T0200264

Nothing to Fear

Nothing to Fear

Demystifying Death
to Live More Fully

Julie McFadden
with Margot Starbuck

Vermilion
LONDON

4

Vermilion, an imprint of Ebury Publishing
20 Vauxhall Bridge Road
London SW1V 2SA

Vermilion is part of the Penguin Random House group of companies
whose addresses can be found at global.penguinrandomhouse.com

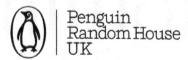

First published in Great Britain by Vermilion in 2024
First published in the United States of America in 2024 by TarcherPerigee,
an imprint of Penguin Random House LLC

The information in this book has been compiled as general guidance on the specific
subjects addressed. It is not a substitute for medical advice. So far as the author
is aware the information given is correct and up to date as at May 2024. Practice,
laws and regulations all change and the reader should obtain up to date professional
advice on any such issues. The author and publishers disclaim, as far as the law
allows, any liability arising directly or indirectly from the use, or misuse,
of the information contained in this book.

www.penguin.co.uk

A CIP catalogue record for this book is available from the British Library

ISBN 9781785045202

Printed and bound in Great Britain by Clays Ltd, Elcograf S.p.A.

The authorised representative in the EEA is Penguin Random House Ireland,
Morrison Chambers, 32 Nassau Street, Dublin D02 YH68

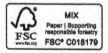

To my patients and their families

Contents

Introduction

Maybe you found me on social media or saw one of my videos about death and dying on the internet. Perhaps you have no idea who I am. Here's what's important as we open this book. My name is Julie, I am a hospice and palliative care nurse, and I want to change the way we look at death and dying.

I've worked as a nurse for over fifteen years now, the first nine years of which were spent working in the intensive care unit (ICU). Later, after I intentionally sought out a career change, I moved to working as a hospice and palliative care nurse. This basically means that every day I work closely with people who are dying or close to death and their families. My hope is to help anticipate and alleviate suffering while optimizing quality of life in these final stages of life. Seeing people die slowly or sometimes unexpectedly in a hospital bed in the ICU made me curious about why we health-care workers weren't having conversations about the end of life with our patients and their families sooner. Seeing both patients and their families experience this kind of shock at the end of life drew me to hospice work.

I knew there had to be a better way to die.

A few years ago, I realized that my unique work as a hospice nurse gave me a level of firsthand experience about death and dying that most people don't know anything about. I'd also seen the contrast between an ICU death and a hospice death, and I recognized that if more people knew what I knew, they would make different end-of-life decisions. In talking with my patients and their families over the years, I realized that I wanted to normalize death by educating people about it in whatever ways I could.

Then, on a trip home to visit my family, I saw my tween nieces making dance videos on TikTok, and I got the idea to start my own TikTok channel about death and dying—a simple place where I could share specialized insights, debunk myths, and tell stories about this topic that seems so taboo in our culture. I started posting a few videos, and before I knew it, I'd gained over a million followers.

Clearly, this content had hit a nerve.

I believe it's deeply important that we educate ourselves about death and dying because we're all going to experience it, one way or another. Most of the time, people either express a fear of death or simply don't want to talk about it at all. Many people don't ever discuss the topic with their loved ones, so death is often a surprise, a shock, resulting in unnecessary suffering. But it doesn't have to be that way.

After personally witnessing hundreds of deaths, I have arrived at a place where I no longer fear the process of dying.

Through my work as a hospice nurse, I've witnessed so many amazing, beautiful, and even miraculous things. I've been with dying people whose eyes fill up with wonder as they tell me they're seeing angels or hearing the most beautiful music they've ever heard. I've seen people's faces light up, smiling big in the moment right before they die. The most miraculous things that I see are the families—the love shared between patients and their families in the moments leading up to death. People who send me messages frequently assume being a hospice nurse is depressing and that witnessing death is sad and terrible, but in so many ways, I find that it's actually the opposite! I get to witness so much love and serve another human being during such a vulnerable time at the end of their life. It's an incredible and sacred gift.

When people are willing to discuss the end of their lives and accept that they're going to die, their whole being changes. They seem to carry with them a special kind of freedom, an attitude that truly helps them live their last days. Their fear decreases, they feel freer, and, ironically, they actually seem more full of life, even though they're dying.

I think this change in perspective can apply to *all* people because, technically, we're all dying. If we can face that fact and allow in a bit of that freedom, I believe we all can live better lives here and now. In this book, I'll share my experiences as a hospice nurse to help readers understand that death isn't something to be feared. Now, it's perfectly normal and natural to feel some fear around death, but even just talking openly about that fear will help loosen the grip it may have on you. I'm going to share some stories and educational resources that I hope will show you that death can be beautiful. If death is normalized and discussed often, we each can walk toward our final days with a lot less fear.

This book isn't necessarily meant to be read from beginning to end. If you want to, you can use the table of contents as your guide. Only you know what you're going through. Perhaps you're caring for someone who is dying, care about someone who is dying, or perhaps you're dying yourself. Pick the topics that are best suited to your situation today. Take what works for you, and leave what doesn't.

A quick disclaimer: I do not officially represent either hospice as an organization or any specific hospice provider. I'm sharing my experience and knowledge with you as I've learned it working with hundreds of hospice patients over the years. Always ask your doctor for the most accurate and up-to-date information. Use the Resources section at the end of this book to get in touch with the right people. Like everything else having to do with your care, ask all the questions and remember that you are the boss.

I hope that, in these pages, you'll discover what I've discovered in my work: that living a life of acceptance helps us live better and die better. Let's take this journey together.

—Hospice Nurse Julie

Chapter 1

The Gift of a Peaceful Death

Before I became a hospice nurse, I worked in the intensive care unit (ICU). In the ICU, doctors and nurses are doing everything possible to keep people alive, and their incredible work saves thousands of lives every year. But we rarely discuss the end of life until it's too late.

People often ask me why I decided to become a hospice nurse. This story is why. I had an ICU patient named Scott who had just had major surgery that was meant to help his advanced-stage pancreatic cancer. I had seen many people get surgeries like Scott's to help extend their lives, and it often worked. In the best cases, successful surgery can add years to a patient's prognosis.

In Scott's case, things went well at first, but after five days, he developed a bilateral pulmonary embolism, which is a blood clot that goes into the lungs and stops blood flow. The only reason he didn't die from this immediately was that he was already in the hospital. Because of this incident, he came back to the ICU.

Scott was intubated, which means he was hooked up to a

machine to help him breathe. As time went on, he would seem to be getting better and even could walk around on his own, but inevitably something bad would happen again. He would be doing really well and then get a blood infection or pneumonia. We just could *not* get him better.

For months, Scott was basically in and out of consciousness. He was on medication to keep his blood pressure normal, and because of the high doses of these meds, his toes turned black. This is called necrosis, and it means the tissue is literally dying. So even if Scott recovered enough to leave the ICU, he would need to have his toes amputated.

Here's the thing: in the ICU, it's all risk versus benefit. We were trying to keep his vitals up no matter what, and sometimes that meant sacrificing comfort and, yes, toes. In the ICU, you have a job to do, and that job is to keep a patient alive at all costs.

As nurses, we were just doing our job. We stayed focused on the numbers that showed how well his kidneys were functioning, how well his liver was functioning, how well his lungs were functioning. We watched these numbers to see which were trending up and which were trending down.

We focused on these minuscule things and reported them to Scott's family, but they had no idea what we were talking about. We would smile and tell them the "creatinine numbers" looked good, but we knew that meant only his kidneys were getting better. However, this information would lead Scott's family to think that eventually everything was going to be better and maybe he would go home one day. But he was still going to die from the cancer, and that wasn't going to change, regardless of how healthy his kidneys became.

This is what we were taught to do in the ICU, and I had become used to situations like this. Our medical team would focus on treating the person, but we were missing the forest for the trees. For a long time, I didn't give this much thought—but watching Scott, I started to think that maybe we had blinders on.

Scott was in the ICU for months. I had developed a good rapport with Scott's family. His wife was always by his side, and she was often anxious and worried. I cared deeply about him and his family. I wanted to speak up, but I was afraid. It was unheard of to have end-of-life discussions with ICU patients and their families. After all, we were supposed to be trying to get them better. But after seeing how much families were suffering, I became convinced we were doing them a disservice. We weren't being honest with them about their loved ones.

One day I finally thought, "Enough is enough." I had seen this pattern in too many patients. I decided to say something during rounds—the daily meetings during which a patient's medical team discusses the patient's care. The head doctor, fellows, residents, medical students, nurses, and patient's family would all be there. I wanted to keep my statements pretty general because I didn't think anyone had told Scott's wife yet that he was dying. *We* knew he wasn't going to get any better, but no one at the hospital would say it.

At rounds, I finally said, "I think we need to have a family meeting to address the bigger picture."

Right away, I knew I had said what everyone had been thinking but couldn't find the words for.

"Yes," everyone agreed, "that's what we need to do."

For the first time in a long time, I felt like I had done something good. I had spoken up and advocated for a patient and their family. It immediately felt right.

That same day, the medical team and the family met with a social worker. The family was given all the facts. Scott had terminal pancreatic cancer. Necrosis had spread to his extremities. Scott was dying. That was the medical reality. But there was another reality, too—the reality that the family had the power to decide how Scott died. They knew him best. They knew how he had lived, and they could give him the gift of a peaceful death if they wished to. With these facts in hand, the family met in private. They decided to remove Scott from the machines that were prolonging his life, and he died later that evening.

Scott's death affected me deeply. It felt strange to advocate for someone's death, even though I knew it was the right thing to do. I felt deeply saddened but empowered at the same time. That was the hardest part. As an ICU nurse, I was committed to treating patients, but something else inside me knew that sometimes it was better to look at the bigger picture. I knew it wasn't right that we kept people in the dark about what was really happening to them. They needed more information, but no one in the ICU was providing it.

People have an incredible capacity for love and compassion. But they need the correct information in order to know when compassion is a better choice than treatment. When we finally did share that information with Scott's family, they finally felt empowered to help Scott die peacefully.

This experience convinced me that, to paraphrase author and podcaster Glennon Doyle, I could do hard things. Speaking up that first time opened up a new world to me, one where I had a voice and could advocate for patients and their families. It convinced me that I could make a difference, even if the end result was the patient dying. I knew in my gut it was the right thing to do, and it gave the family the power to do what they thought was best for their loved one.

I love these patients deeply. I'll never forget them or their families. Speaking up for Scott allowed him to die peacefully, and it profoundly changed the trajectory of my career and my life.

The Difference between the ICU and Hospice

Death in the ICU gets drawn out because, as I mentioned, doctors and nurses are doing everything possible to keep people alive. They're using medications. They're putting people on multiple machines—machines to keep them breathing, machines to filter their blood, machines to work on their kidneys. They're doing surgeries to keep vital organs functioning. That's their focus: preventing death.

To be clear, this is often amazing, life-saving work. But if you really want to know what the inside of an ICU looks like, take a look at the Netflix series *From Scratch*, in which a character named Lino is dying from a rare soft-tissue cancer. A scene in one episode when he's in the ICU felt so much like my experience as an ICU nurse. All the doctors are streaming in and out of his room—the kidney doctor, the liver doctor, the infectious disease doctor—but none of them are talking to each other. The whole time, no one is addressing the fact that Lino has terminal cancer—because that is the oncologist's job.

That is exactly what really happens, and it's exactly why I left the ICU. Unfortunately, in the medical system we work within, it's difficult for providers to communicate with each other. We're taught to work within our own little bubble. Because I've been there, I know what the staff are thinking. They're thinking, "Well, maybe I'm not right. Maybe the oncologist knows something I don't know. Maybe they know something that hasn't been relayed to me." So no one says anything.

And when no one says anything, it can get really ugly. I've seen patients lose limbs because we were using meds that squeezed their arteries and veins to keep their blood pressure up, cutting off blood supply in their extremities in the process. When your goal is to keep someone alive, keeping the blood pumping through their veins is more important than losing a limb.

But the truth is, some of the people in the ICU are going to die no matter what treatments they receive, yet we still work to keep everyone alive at all costs. Period. This all-or-nothing kind of thinking is everywhere, and it's not the fault of one person; *it's the culture*. What I am advocating for is injecting more information into the process so that families are prepared and empowered to make the right decisions for their loved ones—rather than defaulting to measures like amputation because they don't know there are any other options.

We are fortunate enough to live in a country that already has a solution to address this cultural blind spot. It's called hospice, and it's a program that helps terminally ill people live better. After my experience with Scott in the ICU, I made a change. I became a hospice nurse and started down a new path.

Preparing for Death

Many people assume that dying is the worst possible outcome. But that's not always the case. Watching someone suffer or endure a poor quality of life for an extended period of time is far worse, in my opinion. Yet many of us look at death as the worst thing that can happen to us. We'll do anything to stop it, and because of that, we create unnecessary suffering for ourselves and for our loved ones.

I saw that up close during my years as an ICU nurse. I've seen what it looks like when our health-care system doesn't allow someone to die peacefully. Hospital staff are just following procedures. They're not doing anything wrong, but they're doing everything to keep someone alive.

We have such a fear of death that we panic. Maybe we're the person who is dying, and we fear death. Maybe we're a loved one who's trying to help someone else go through it. Or we may even be that medical professional who was trained to keep people alive at all costs. But we can cause a lot of unnecessary suffering when we don't know how to stop, when we don't know how to let go—or maybe when we don't realize that we *can* let go.

So let's begin thinking about it differently: What if death isn't the worst possible outcome? How would that change the way we live our lives and treat the illnesses that we have? What if we value quality over quantity? Let's get curious.

What if death isn't the worst possible outcome?

What a Peaceful Death Looks Like

Rosa and Pedro were in their forties with two young children. Pedro was dying of cancer, and Rosa was taking care of him. I was their hospice nurse, visiting their home two or three times a week. They spoke only Spanish, and I had to use an interpreter to communicate with them, but Rosa and I became so close that I often forgot there was someone on the phone translating for us. I seemed to understand her through her eyes. We formed a deep connection.

Pedro's young age and the presence of the children made the situation especially difficult. His family was struggling, but the love in the house was palpable. The love overtook the sadness. I'll never forget this family because of the deep, deep sense of love I felt there. I got to see love in action.

In the last days of Pedro's life, the house was filled with

family and friends. The day that Pedro died, I was there. Rosa's head was resting on his chest. She was gently speaking to him in Spanish. Both Pedro's and Rosa's parents were there also, circled around the bed, loving him, honoring him, and caring for him. Pedro's parents rubbed his head. Everyone surrounded him, saying wonderful, loving things and supporting this man as he took his last breath. You could *feel* the love.

This is what a prepared death looks like.

Since leaving the ICU and moving into hospice care, I now get to truly *serve* patients who are dying. Unlike the scramble to keep people alive in the ICU, when people who are dying have the choice to *prepare* for death, they can experience a *peaceful* death.

My friend Ashley Bryant, a death doula and the founder of Distant Shores Deathcare, uses this analogy: Imagine you're on a beach with the ocean in front of you. The ocean is death. Will you get pulled into the ocean via the undertow, against your will, kicking and screaming? Or do you cross this ocean in a boat you made, with your friends and family beside you, shoving the boat off and sailing of your own accord? That is the difference between a prepared death and an unprepared one.

Everyone has an end-of-life journey, but when you're on hospice, you get to embrace yours. It's not quite "borrowed" time, but you do have a kind of gift that people who die suddenly do not have. When you know you're dying, you get to make a plan. You get to grow into acceptance around it. You get to tell your family and friends you love them. You get to plan visits with them.

The more you let go and accept that you're dying, the better you'll live while you're still alive. The more peace you make with the idea of your death, the more peacefully you'll exit this world. And the better prepared you are for your death, the better prepared your family will be for your death. When you prepare— by facing your death squarely, by getting your financial things figured out, by making your funeral arrangements—you are caring for your family. When you ready yourself for death, you don't have to suffer in pain. You get to ask for help. You get to celebrate and *live* the days you have.

I mentioned that the death of Pedro, who was physically comfortable and surrounded by loved ones, was a beautiful and peaceful death. But I've also witnessed those who've died differently.

I cared for a woman named Martha in the ICU. She had a terminal cancer diagnosis but had come into the hospital for an extensive surgery that was meant to extend her life. Unfortunately, she, like Scott, kept having complications during her hospital stay that would land her back with me in the ICU for months. By her sixth month in the ICU, her toes and fingers were necrotic, and she was fully dependent on machines to keep her alive. The ICU team began having family meetings to discuss the reality of the situation: we were keeping her alive, and the likelihood of her "getting better" was extremely low. But her family refused, time and time again, to turn off the machines and allow her to die peacefully.

Even with the machines, Martha began to decline and had to be resuscitated with chest compressions several times. Again, despite us explaining how much Martha was likely suffering, the family could not let her go. The hospital eventually had to bring in the ethics committee to explain why turning off the machines and allowing Martha to die peacefully was the ethical choice. Even after that, the family was resistant. It was just a sad, awful death for everyone involved.

As you think about the type of death you'd choose, imagine standing on that shore and choosing between those two ways to die. Martha's experience was more like getting swept out to sea against your will, struggling all the while. The other option, the one Pedro chose, is the one where he got to cross that ocean in a boat that he lovingly made with his friends and family. After saying their goodbyes, they cast off the boat and Pedro sailed off of his own volition.

A peaceful death can look many different ways.

There are certain signs when someone is actively dying, which I'll discuss in more detail in chapter 5—changes in breathing, skin color, temperature, and so on—and we can witness those even when someone is experiencing a peaceful death. Although some of these signals may feel foreign to us, they're a normal part of the process of natural death. They're not causing the person who is dying discomfort.

When people who are dying, and their families, accept the interventions that hospice offers, those more distressing symptoms are rarely seen in the final stage when a person is actively dying.

Here are some examples of what to look for:

PEACEFUL DEATH	UNPEACEFUL DEATH
• Pain and/or other symptoms, if present, are managed. • End-of-life wishes have been discussed and written out. • The person is clean, safe, and comfortable. • The person has all the support they need.	• Pain and/or symptoms are not managed. • The person is not clean, safe, and comfortable. • The person does not have the support they need. • The family is refusing to let the dying person go.

A person who is in the early stages of their journey toward death, who is still alert and oriented, can continue to make choices that allow for a peaceful death until the very end. They can be clean, safe, and comfortable. They can be free of pain. They can invite the people who mean the most to them to be present. They can create the environment they need to die peacefully.

When they're no longer alert and oriented, those around the dying person can take over. They can surround the person with loving care. They can create a positive mood in the room with lighting, music, and gentle touch. They can speak gentle words of love and affirmation. That's what Pedro's family did.

What's worse than death is a death that's resisted, painful, or chaotic. But a peaceful death? A good death? It's what each of us deserves.

Many Times

Maribel hadn't married and didn't have any children. Although she'd had many friends who loved her dearly, at the age of 102, just about everyone she'd known throughout her life was dead. At the end, Maribel had a caregiver, and she had me.

During one of my last visits, her caregiver and I sat together looking through Maribel's photo albums and talking about how wonderful she was. As I reflected on her life that had lasted over a century, I wanted to make sure I'd understood correctly that she'd never been married, even for a short time. Although she'd been unresponsive all day, I suspected she could still hear me, so I asked, "Maribel, were you ever married?"

Matter-of-factly, she answered, "No."

"Maribel," I continued, "were you ever in love?"

Eyes closed, in a weak voice, and with some attitude, Maribel answered with certainty: "Many times."

The caregiver and I just laughed. *Hell yeah.* I knew that others might see a 102-year-old woman dying without being surrounded by family and friends as tragic. But with those two words—"many times"—I knew that despite the absence of children and grandchildren in that moment, there wasn't sadness in that house. Maribel had lived a rich, beautiful life with parents, siblings, friends, and lovers who just weren't in the room. And although I can't anticipate exactly what the afterlife will be like, I couldn't help but imagine Maribel drifting off to sleep and waking up surrounded by all these people she's missed for a long time.

Embracing the Sacredness of Death

I am asked all the time why in the world I would do something as difficult as working for hospice. People often ask, "Isn't it so depressing?" It's sad sometimes, yes. There's really no way around that. But I don't find my job to be depressing. In a way, it's actually a sacred gift to me. This is one of the reasons that sharing the stories of the prepared deaths I've experienced is so important to me. The people I've met in their dying moments have changed my outlook on life, and far from depressing, I find them precious and inspiring.

Take Jason, eighty, married, with children and grandchildren. When he was diagnosed with metastatic liver cancer and it was clear that he was in his final days of life, his whole family gathered in the home where he and his wife, Susan, had raised their children.

I had been Jason's hospice nurse for a few weeks, and his condition, although terminal, remained stable. The last time I made a visit, however, his condition had changed.

In the couple's bedroom, Jason was unconscious and unresponsive. Jason and Susan's three children and several grandchildren were gathered around his bed, thumbing through a stack of photo albums. They were laughing and crying as each of them shared their favorite family stories and memories: trips to the lake, Christmas and holiday highlights, secret childhood mischief. The love surrounding Jason was everything anyone could ask for as they moved toward death.

Wanting to honor that time but also be available for whatever they needed, I stationed myself in an office space across the hall to record my notes about the visit. As I worked, I heard snippets of the family's conversation.

"We love you, Dad. We love you."

"It's so easy to love you."

"You've been the best husband."

"It's okay. You can let go."

"We love you."

The entire family had transitioned effortlessly with Jason's sudden decline and were able to say goodbye the way they wanted. To me in the other room, it felt like a powerful, sacred love. It felt, ironically, like this type of death is what life is supposed to be all about.

What I do doesn't feel depressing because I see patients have these beautiful deaths, being welcomed in love to a place that's *good*. I get to witness families and friends really loving each other well. I get to help people who are dying feel comfortable as they die and help them and their loved ones embrace the reality of death—which helps them live better *and* die better. I see the power in what is possible as we faithfully accompany people toward death. As professionals, and as loved ones, we have the power to make a real difference in people's lives.

If you're one of those people who assumes that accompanying people on their death journeys is depressing, I hope this book will open your eyes to something new.

Chapter 2

Death Is Not a Dirty Word

One of the reasons we find death so frightening is that a lot of us refuse to talk about it. We've made it such a taboo topic, I think half of the fear we feel is just from *avoiding* it. Avoiding talking about it. Avoiding learning about it. If we did those things, it'd be less scary. The more willing someone is to talk about and accept the fact of their death, the better they'll live, and the better they'll die.

You've heard the way people talk about someone who's died.

"She's gone."

"He's no longer with us."

"They passed on."

I get it. It's gentler. But as we think about shifting the way we look at death and dying, we also need to look at the words we use and start getting comfortable with saying the words: he's *dying*, she's *dead*, they *died*.

Death.

I understand that not everyone's there yet. But we all can start trying it on a little bit. Try saying, "Mom died." Try saying,

"I'm dying." Try saying those words; it's actually really therapeutic. Plus, by using them yourself, you give others permission to use the "d-words," too.

Specifically, I think it's important to talk about death with the person who is dying, when they're lucid. I see that my patients who are willing to talk about their death and what they want before they die have more peaceful lives and far more peaceful deaths. It helps their loved ones, too. Often I'll begin, "We all have an end-of-life journey. All of us. Right now, yours is a little clearer than other people's. So what is that going to look like?" Then I talk about death and dying. When I model doing it, the patients and their family members are usually a little more comfortable talking about it themselves.

We All Have an End-of-Life Journey

One of the ways I like to ease people into this conversation is by beginning, "We all have an end-of-life journey . . ." Because we do. Once I've broken the ice, I begin to speak more freely about death and dying. When you're comfortable talking about death, you give others permission to be comfortable talking about death, too.

Some people ask me, "Why is it so important for people to know that they're going to die?" It's a great question. When people choose to learn about their particular illness and what their death might look like, their fears often are eased as they acknowledge what's happening. The people who are willing to discuss end-of-life issues and to accept that they're going to die seem to carry about them a certain type of freedom, and they truly live their last days well. Their fear tends to decrease, and they tend to be freer and more full of life, even though they're dying.

I've also seen the opposite. When people are unwilling to look squarely at death, the last few months of their life are usually filled with fear, anxiety, and stress. There seems to be a lot of existential suffering and chaos. That's why I want to normalize talk about death and dying and spread the understanding that we're all going to die. (And as I mentioned in the introduction, I think this can apply to all people, not just the actively dying, because we're *all* technically dying!)

Demolishing the Taboos

One of the reasons I'm so passionate about educating people about death and dying is because I've seen firsthand how our culture sanitizes the topic.

We hide it.

We embalm it.

We put makeup on it.

We photoshop it.

We don't say the d-word.

We get a babysitter for the kids while we attend a funeral.

And even if we do allow the body of a person who's died to be viewed at a funeral or memorial service, we make 100 percent sure that it looks as *alive* as possible.

When we break the taboos around facing and discussing death, we also break the power of fear around it.

If you feel scared of death—if you don't even want to think about it or talk about it—I have really good news for you: *you are totally normal*. But I want to change what *normal* is. I want conversations about death to happen, even if they're uncomfortable—*especially* if they're uncomfortable. That's one reason I started a TikTok channel where I talk about death and dying. Social media eases the conversation in a way that makes people feel safe.

Most people think they don't want to talk about death. But here's what I'll tell you: after they get introduced to it, they're on board. I receive hundreds of messages from people who have watched my stories online telling me that I've helped them with their death anxiety. Learning about death and understanding it a little more has eased their fear.

That's exactly why I want to help everyone understand what's happening at the end of life. Because we've largely avoided death so successfully, we don't understand what we're seeing when we *are* near death. The most natural process in the world, which every one of us will face, feels foreign to us. I'm convinced that it doesn't have to be this way.

If you haven't spent time around people who are dying, you may feel anxious about being on hospice, having a loved one on hospice, and death in general. If you're seeing things you haven't seen before and hearing sounds you haven't heard before, you may be wondering, "Should that happen? Is that normal? Are they suffering?" This can be confusing and even scary. In this book, I want you to discover what a body looks like when it's dying. What it sounds like. What it feels like. What it smells like. When we break the taboos around facing and discussing death, we also break the power of fear around it. As we begin to understand death and become more comfortable with it, we can not only *die* better, but also *live* better.

As we begin to understand death and become more comfortable with it, we can not only die better, but also live better.

On the other hand, when we're intimidated by fear, when we refuse to face death, we forfeit our choice to shape the kind of death we'll experience. I hope that you'll begin to notice and own all the choices you can make to embrace a peaceful death. Being able to look at and speak about death has demonstrable benefits, not just for our dying but also for our living. That has certainly been my experience as I've been with people on their journeys toward death. I've learned from these precious patients what matters most. They've taught me to enjoy my loved ones. To savor each day. To live life on purpose.

So I'm inviting you to consider a revolutionary possibility: dying is not the worst possible outcome. What would be different if we truly accepted this truth? What would be different about the way we lived out our days? What would be different about the way we died? I want to suggest that *everything* would be different. When we're willing to face death, we can live—and die—well.

The Language We Use

If we're ever going to deal with death openly, the first thing we need to learn how to do is to talk about it. It's evident in the language we use that we're uncomfortable discussing death:

"Mom passed."

"He's gone."

"She's in a better place."

"God wanted her with him."

"There's another angel in heaven."

A first step in changing our attitudes toward death is to use words that are honest. Practice saying these phrases, or your personal version of them, aloud:

"They're dying soon."

"She died."

"He is dead."

"I am dying."

I know that last one is rough. I know it takes courage. But there's value in speaking what is most real. It's therapeutic. That's why I'm giving you permission to use all the d-words: *death, died, dead, dying.*

Sometimes it's hard for people to accept that they're dying. I often hear:

"I don't want to think I'm dying."

"This is not happening."

"I don't want to act like I'm dying."

"I'm not dying."

"I don't want to leave my spouse."

"I don't want to leave my children."

These sentences are hard to read, let alone say out loud. But what I know is if we refuse to face the reality of a diagnosis, we do a disservice to ourselves and those around us. And the converse is also true. When we're able to face what's coming with realism and still have hope, we can make the best choices about our living and our dying.

Let's say we know that someone at a particular stage of a particular disease has about six months to live. We often have a pretty good idea of how those six months will unfold. So I ask questions like these:

"What do you want these six months to look like?"

"Do you want to be at home with your family?"

"Do you want good pain management? And symptom management?"

And I'll always add something like, "You don't have to make a choice today. But I want you to think about it. If these are your last six months, how do you want them to be? You get to decide."

Permission Granted

Many people feel as though they have to use every means necessary, for as long as possible, to keep themselves or their loved one alive. The person who is dying also may have this impulse. I understand why it's tempting. But if you or your loved one is in the process of dying, I want to give you permission to allow the dying process to happen.

Josephine and Sylvia

How we communicate about death, the words we use, and the attitudes we adopt all play a huge role in helping the actively dying and their loved ones accept death and prepare for it. I want to share the stories of two women, Josephine and Sylvia, to show you just how much the words we use—and the words we don't use—matter.

First, Josephine. She was in her mid-eighties when she entered hospice. When her doctor diagnosed her with metastatic cancer about a month earlier, she'd made it clear that Josephine likely had less than six months to live.

When I arrived at Josephine's house to admit her to hospice, she was not particularly warm and fuzzy. That's okay! Everybody's personality is different. I take that into account when I'm working with a patient. In this case, I kept to the business at hand: admission. This means some paperwork, lots of questions, taking vitals, and determining the best level of care for the patient. By the end of the visit, which lasted about an hour, Josephine definitely had started warming up to me. She relaxed and laid down on the couch, her hands behind her head, something clearly on her mind. I thought perhaps she had something she wanted to share, but because she was a quiet person, I didn't probe. Instead, I lingered a little longer and made it clear with my open body language that I was available to her if she wanted to talk.

After some time, Josephine said, "I'm not scared of death. But I'm curious. I wonder what it's going to be like to take my last breath. I've been a Christian my whole life. I truly believe there is a God. I just wonder, when I take my last breath, am I going to open my eyes and see God?"

As she said this, her eyes teared up. It wasn't my impression that she was sad, just that she was feeling the importance of what she'd been thinking. I so wanted to be able to answer her, to tell her everything would be all right, to tell her she would see just what she wanted to see. But I couldn't. It wasn't easy. I think we all have an urge to make it better with words, but really what's needed is connection. So I didn't say a word. Not a word. I just sat there and listened to her talk because that's what Josephine needed most right then. We breathed together, and my own eyes welled up a little, too.

When she was done, we looked into each other's eyes. I sighed and said the truth: "I don't know. But I guess we'll see."

And then we laughed. We laughed hard, and it felt amazing.

And that was that. That was the whole conversation. After that, I knew that Josephine was prepared, even though we hadn't spoken all that much. I felt a beautiful connection to her, and I knew that ultimately, I had helped her by just listening to her, seeing her, and not trying or pretending to have all the answers. It helped me, too. There's something so human for me there. I love connecting with people like that. We don't need all the answers; we just need to speak the truth. When we can talk about death, when we make space for it, we are able to face it squarely.

The second story I want to share with you is about Sylvia. Sylvia came onto hospice in her early sixties, also with metastatic cancer. She and her family clearly had not been given full and accurate information about either hospice or death. They reported to me that they'd been told hospice "offered extra services" in the home to help with pain management. This is true. But no one had told Sylvia or her family members that part of the criteria—in fact, the most important part of the criteria—for receiving hospice care is that the patient has less than six months to live. So even though they'd signed up for hospice care, they had no idea that she was dying. The fact that Sylvia had metastatic disease was all throughout her medical chart . . . yet she still was listed as "full code," meaning that she wanted everything possible to be done to revive her if her heart and lungs stopped working. (I'll discuss codes more in chapter 7.)

When I first met Sylvia, knowing what I know as a hospice nurse, it was clear to me that she was dying. She was on high-flow oxygen. She was huffing and puffing. She couldn't speak. What was even clearer to me was that nobody else in her life had the slightest idea that Sylvia was going to die. Soon.

I invited Sylvia and her family to have a conversation with me. In this instance, there was much to say.

We all pulled some kitchen chairs into Sylvia's bedroom, and I began to share. "Everyone has an end-of-life journey. Let's talk about *your* end-of-life journey."

As the words came out of my mouth, I could see on every single face that I'd introduced something they hadn't yet heard or understood. The confusion that washed across their expressions told me what I already suspected: they didn't know that Sylvia was at the end of her life. *How was that even possible? How did someone get this far in their disease and not know that yet?*

They ended up calling 911 and she ultimately died in the hospital, just two days later.

Sylvia and her family had been kept in the dark. I don't want to blame this situation on specific providers because I don't know what they said. But I do believe that when patients don't receive the information they need to hear in the way they need to hear it, our health-care system is failing people and robbing them of the chance to experience peaceful deaths. I learned in the ICU that someone who doesn't know they're dying will continue to accept the interventions we offer—interventions that *we* know won't save them from death—because they believe these procedures will "keep them from dying." What a disservice we're doing to patients like Sylvia.

Whatever Sylvia's doctor had *said* to her and the family, what was undeniable was that they hadn't *received* the information they needed to make the best decisions about her end-of-life journey. I believe that one of the main factors driving poor communication like this is a discomfort in our culture around speaking about death and dying.

Josephine had the opportunity—and the willingness—to thoughtfully consider her death and arrive at a place where she felt not scared of death but curious about it; Sylvia did not. What was the difference between them? Of course, every person is an individual, and every end-of-life journey is unique. Josephine and Sylvia had different communication styles and needs. But the main difference was that one received honest communication about death, and one didn't.

Honesty Matters

Being honest about death matters because it's the right thing to do—but also because there are real consequences to consider. When we refuse to talk about death, we rob people of the ability to make informed choices about how they live and how they die.

When I talk to people with terminal diagnoses who are resisting death, I try to help them see they have options. I had a conversation like this recently with a father in his early forties who was dying.

"The only advice I can give you," I explained, "is to hope for the best and plan for the worst. We know that someone with your disease is likely to die within six months. So how do you want those last six months to look? Do you want to be at home with your family, doing the things you want to do, with good pain management and symptom management and doctors and nurses coming to you? Or would you like to continue aggressive and potentially uncomfortable or debilitating treatments that may or may not buy you a little more quantity of time?"

He was willing to hear that and thanked me for saying it.

I added, "You don't have to make a choice today. But I just want you to think about it. How do you want to live if this is your last six months?"

The choice truly is the patient's, but they only know they even *have* a choice if they hear both sides of the story. I think you can tell which side of the argument I fall on. In my experience, continuing treatment despite a terminal diagnosis brings suffering and discomfort and, in fact, rarely extends life to any meaningful degree. I've seen this in the ICU, and I've seen this in hospice, and it's a huge part of the reason I'm writing this book (and hopefully a huge part of the reason you're reading it).

I'm not saying honesty about death is always easy. It's not. Letting someone know that continued treatments won't save their life and may not even extend it—in fact, may possibly shorten it—is a super hard truth to say to someone. But it's what needs to be said. I understand that we often don't want to say the really hard truths, but I think that's unfair to the patient.

I've seen too often in hospitals that no one is willing to have the hard conversations about death and dying. I've been with patients who ended up in the hospital and were diagnosed with a terminal illness, yet no one had taken the time to make that plain to them. They knew that they were sick, but they didn't understand that they would die within six to twelve months. They didn't know they had a terminal illness. I wish this was rare, but it's not.

To be clear, I don't think any medical professional ever means to do a disservice to patients. Everyone is doing their best. But in our flawed health-care system, doctors and nurses don't have the time to fully talk with patients. They're taught to be focused and quick. No one is ever purposely trying to lie to patients, but sometimes when they do deliver the bad news, it's simply not intelligible. They say things like this:

"I'm sorry to tell you this, but statistically, this isn't a diagnosis that proves to have longevity."

"Outcomes are poor."

"We've done everything we can do."

In case you didn't pick it up, when you hear these words from a doctor, you've likely just been told you're dying.

Sometimes these pronouncements are quickly followed by treatment options:

"But here's what we can do for you . . ."

"These are things we can do that may help you live longer . . ."

"We've seen some good results with . . ."

And although doctors absolutely should make sure you know what all the options are, I need you to know that those options don't always change the fact that you are dying. And in the case of diagnoses that likely are terminal, you will fare best when you're able to be realistic about what's ahead.

Follow Up

When doctors deliver an initial diagnosis, one that is likely to be terminal, it's a lot of information for a patient to process. It's natural for a patient to experience a degree of shock that makes it difficult to hear anything that comes after a word like *cancer.* If this happens to you, return for a follow-up appointment, and bring a journal, a recorder, or someone you trust so you can absorb the rest of the news about treatments, outcomes, and so forth.

Medical professionals who have to deliver difficult news to patients are human. We're not superheroes. We're just like you.

We wish the news was better.

We don't want to say the hard words.

We want to soften the blow.

We don't want to dash the patient's hopes.

Yet the kindest thing that patients can receive is the truth. When patients have all the information about their condition, they can make the best choices about how to live more freely and die how they choose.

When patients have all the information about their condition, they can make the best choices about how to live more freely and die how they choose.

I think some doctors believe they're keeping hope alive when they sidestep hard conversations. I totally agree that hope matters. I understand that sometimes patients aren't ready to hear such huge news, and as medical professionals we have to do our best to meet them where they are. But I also think that patients are *entitled* to have the best information about their health and that it *serves* them the best. The more a patient can anticipate the likely outcome of their condition, the better they can live the rest of their lives, hoping for the best but preparing for the worst. But if the patient doesn't know that they should be preparing for the worst, we've done them—we've done *you*—a disservice.

Although it shouldn't be all on you, you can ask your doctor to share with you what you need to know about your disease. For instance, if I were ever diagnosed with a terminal condition, I'd say, "I'd like you to speak candidly about my prognosis. I want to know what typically happens."

It breaks my heart when I see patients with multiple hospital admissions who are battling a disease that medical professionals know is terminal but the patients haven't yet understood that. They'll spend all their money, even going into debt, to fight what will not be a winning battle.

Talking about the D-word

One of the most gracious things you can do when you or your loved one is dying is to make room for conversations about death, especially if, as a family member, you have information from care providers that the person who is dying is not yet privy

How to Communicate
with Maximum Clarity

This script can be a guide for communicating with your doctor
with maximum clarity:

- **Give permission.** "I welcome you to speak candidly
  with me."
- **Ask about the likely progression.** "I'm interested in
  knowing the likely progression and outcome of this
  disease."
- **Inquire about treatment options.** "I'm interested
  to know if there are treatment options that have
  proven effective."
- **Ask about hospice.** "I'd like to know if it would be
  better not to pursue treatments. Is there a point at
  which you may suggest hospice care?"

If your doctor still avoids the issue, you also could try asking,
point blank, "If your mother had this, what would you recommend? If it were *you*, what would you do?"

to. Exceptions to this are instances of confusion or dementia. If
your loved one is experiencing diminished mental capacity, it's
best to consult with your medical professionals about what level
of communication is recommended. For most people, however,
when they know that they are dying, it's best if they have the opportunity to talk about it. When they can talk about death, they

have the opportunity to normalize it. When they normalize it, they have the opportunity to accept it.

To take it even further, the person who can learn about how they will die—whether from amyotrophic lateral sclerosis (ALS), cancer, or something else—is at an even greater advantage. Having the best information really can ease their fears and prepare them to weather what's coming with a greater degree of awareness and comfort. I see a beautiful freedom in these folks who've been bold and brave enough to face the reality of their situation. Although they're technically dying, these individuals truly *live* in their last days.

Conversely, my experience has shown me that a person who is *not* offered the opportunity to face their death squarely is at a great disadvantage. The individual who resists acknowledging their death by refusing to talk about it or learn about it likely will have a death that is anything but peaceful. At the end of their lives, these individuals often are racked with fear, anxiety, and stress. Even beyond the physical experience, these "resisters" more often experience an existential suffering as well.

Death is not a dirty word, and in case you're worried, I can tell you that simply talking about it is not going to make it happen any faster. But talking about it *can* help you or your loved one be better prepared for what to expect. And it can help you loosen the grip of the perfectly natural fear we all feel at first when contemplating death.

Furthermore, it's not just dying people who need to think about and talk about death. Whether you've been diagnosed with a terminal illness or not, everyone benefits when they're able to consider their own death. That's why I encourage everyone to think about what they would and wouldn't want when they die. What they'd want if they could no longer swallow. Whether they'd want cardiopulmonary resuscitation (CPR) at the end. Whether they'd want to be intubated. Even what they'd want at their funeral. (I'll go into more detail about all these options in chapter 7.) If you're willing to have these conversations now, whoever you are, it will help immensely in your future.

Chapter 3

How Hospice Helps

S o what is hospice? Hospice is care for people at the end of life—that is, people who have a terminal diagnosis and a life expectancy of six months or less. Specifically, hospice offers person-centered care to address physical, emotional, and spiritual needs at the end of life. Hospice lets a dying person live out their remaining days as well as they possibly can and then die as well as they possibly can.

Hospice can help you avoid the hospital so that you can spend the time you have left doing the things that are meaningful to you. It can help you stay wherever it is that you call home so that you can be surrounded by family and friends. If you don't have a home or prefer not to be there, some states offer hospice-care facilities, often with a very homelike feel.

People who are eligible for hospice care are terminally ill; *they are dying*. That means that whether or not they choose to go on hospice, they will die. If the dying person has symptoms related to a disease, hospice will treat those symptoms, but hospice neither speeds up nor slows down a person's death. What hospice does is help people die more peacefully, by allowing the natural process of dying to happen.

Hospice Care
versus Palliative Care

Hospice care and palliative care are closely related, but they're not quite the same thing. Like hospice care, palliative care involves comfort-focused symptom management for people who have a serious illness. Unlike hospice care, it's provided to patients who aren't necessarily expected to die in the next six months. Palliative care patients can continue treatments for the disease if they want (for example, they can keep receiving chemo if they have cancer), whereas hospice patients stop treatment.

Likely Candidates for Hospice Care

Certain conditions may make a person a likely candidate to receive hospice care. This is very general because even with these diagnoses, treatment options may be available. However, broadly speaking, certain cancer diagnoses and other chronic terminal illnesses often end up in hospice care. Some of the most common ones include the following:

Cancers

- Pancreatic cancer

- Metastatic cancer to multiple parts of the body

- Glioblastoma

- Cholangiocarcinoma, or bile duct cancer

Terminal chronic illnesses

- End-stage kidney disease

- Liver disease

- Heart disease, such as congestive heart failure

- Lung disease, such as chronic obstructive pulmonary disease (COPD)

- Amyotrophic lateral sclerosis (ALS)

- Brain diseases, like Alzheimer's

Eight Facts to Know about Hospice

Even if you have a general understanding about what hospice care is, if you haven't experienced it, you may not know much about the details. Here are eight of the most important facts to know about hospice care:

1. **Hospice care can extend life.** Studies have demonstrated that, among people with identical conditions that are no longer being treated, those receiving hospice care live longer.

2. **Hospice care is (usually) free.** Hospice is a benefit covered by Medicare, Medicaid, and most private health insurances. So those receiving hospice care don't usually need to pay out of pocket.

3. **Hospice care is offered for diseases other than cancer.** Hospice is not just for people with cancer. Those with other chronic, terminal illnesses can qualify. (A terminal illness means a prognosis of six months or less to live.)

4. **Hospice care most often happens at home.** Most hospice care occurs in your home. Sometimes a person may be in a hospice facility, though; this varies from state to state and patient to patient.

5. **Hospice care gives you more control, not less.** When you're in hospice, you call the shots. Everything is designed to make your remaining life more comfortable. Because aggressive treatments have been discontinued, you get to determine how much or little care you want to receive.

6. **Hospice care doesn't disqualify you from seeking regular medical care.** Signing up for hospice doesn't mean that you lose all your benefits. You still can see

doctors who are unrelated to the diagnosis that qualified
you to receive hospice care.

7. **Hospice care can be stopped by you at any time.** You
   can change your mind at any time, going off hospice care
   whenever you choose. You also can switch providers if
   you'd like.

8. **Hospice care offers services to your family as well.**
   Hospice providers not only care for the patient, but also
   offer services to family members. Social workers and
   chaplains who work with patients also can work with
   family members, and bereavement services are usually
   available for up to a year after the patient dies.

The Five Biggest Myths about Hospice

The biggest misconception about hospice is that we kill people.
Let me be 100 percent clear: *hospice does not kill people.* When
people come on hospice, they are already terminally ill. That
means they are already going to die. Hospice provides the care
they need to live well before they die and then to die well when
they finally do.

Let's take a look at a few more myths about hospice:

1. **"Hospice just pushes morphine, causing people to
   die faster."**
   Fact: *Although we do offer morphine for pain relief, studies
   show that people who receive hospice care live longer than*

those who do not. I've heard the theory that hospice "wants people dead," the idea being that the more people who die on hospice, the more money hospice companies will make. Actually, the opposite is true! The more people who stay on hospice—that is, the more people who remain alive—the more money the companies make. But to be clear, we're not in your home to maximize profit. We're there because we want to help and serve you.

2. **"People don't get any kind of treatment or care on hospice."**
    Fact: *Contrary to popular belief, we don't just stop all treatment. Actually, we treat all kinds of conditions that patients may be dealing with. We just don't offer treatments for the disease that is taking their lives. For example, when you're receiving hospice care for metastatic colon cancer, you won't be seeing your oncologist. You won't be receiving chemo treatments or radiation. You won't be seeing doctors who have anything to do with your terminal diagnosis. But if you have heart issues in addition to the cancer diagnosis, you can see your cardiologist. We can also run labs, tests, or procedures if the results will help manage your symptoms—for example, get a PleurX drainage tube placed to help manage ascites. We're always working to provide the best quality of life for each patient.*

3. **"Hospice dehydrates or starves people to death."**
    Fact: *We never withhold food or hydration that the patient wants and needs. A hospice patient can have as much or as*

*little food and drink as they want whenever they want it.
People at the end of life often refuse food and liquid, choosing
not to eat or drink, and we honor that. That's because we
know that a dying body is not a hungry body or a thirsty
body. (More on this in chapter 5.)*

4. **"Hospice care only happens in the final few days of
   a person's life."**
   Fact: *Hospice is truly about living, and some people have been
   receiving hospice care for years. We are always working to
   genuinely provide quality of life. Unfortunately, I have heard
   some doctors recommend, "Don't go on hospice until the very
   end." This is terrible advice. Go on hospice when you're ready
   to go on hospice! If you have a life-limiting illness and are no
   longer receiving treatments, go on hospice. If you ever feel like
   you want to try another treatment or procedure, you can just
   come off hospice. You're not "stuck" on hospice once you sign
   on. Hospice is only here to help you. We can provide care to
   make the time you have left better, whether that's five months
   or five days.*

5. **"Hospice providers offer twenty-four-hour
   care."**
   Fact: *In addition to regularly scheduled visits from your
   hospice nurse, all agencies have a twenty-four-hour-care
   hotline that you can call and request a nurse visit at any
   hour. However, this nurse will only help with the pressing
   issue, such as pain. She won't stay around the clock.*

Unfortunately, hospice does not provide day-to-day care or custodial care. What we do, however, is teach families how best to care for their loved one who is dying. In very rare cases that meet specific guidelines, Medicare can authorize continuous care.

We're Here to Help

Lynn was in her late fifties and dying of ALS. Her daughter and primary caregiver, Gina, was only in her early twenties. It was just the two of them, and like a lot of the families I serve, this pair was just so easy to love. Although Lynn was alert mentally, she was struggling physically. She was no longer able to swallow, she was producing lots of excess secretions, and she was beginning to have trouble breathing (unfortunately, common symptoms with ALS). Her daughter was giving her subcutaneous medication to help with these issues, but Lynn still seemed really uncomfortable. Most heartbreaking was that she'd lost her ability to communicate. (Some people with ALS learn to communicate using a computer program that can read their eye movements, but Lynn had not.)

Sometimes the hospice agency provided a twenty-four-hour-care nurse, but as soon as Lynn's symptoms improved, the nurse would be taken off her case. Invariably, Lynn's symptoms would get worse again, and Gina would have to pick up the slack. At the end of each day, Gina was physically exhausted and emotionally at her wits' end. Each time Lynn would lose that nurse, I'd fight harder to get her back again. I worked for a great company, but they had to follow Medicare's strict rules and regulations about what could be provided to families.

I remember one afternoon outside the home, screaming at my boss on the phone, "You're not here! I am! I'm telling you, we need this and we need it now!" Then I started sobbing. Thankfully, I won, and Lynn received the care she needed. She died peacefully at home, with her daughter at her side.

I don't share this story to make myself out as some kind of hero. But if you're unfamiliar with hospice, I want you to know that *we're here to help*. We're here to fight for you, and we'll do everything we can to make your death as peaceful and comfortable as possible.

Hospice-Care FAQs

When people start considering hospice care, a few questions tend to come up. I'll answer some of the most frequently asked questions in this section.

When Is It Time for Hospice?

Much of our health-care system is built around treating disease. It takes a real change in mindset for a health-care professional—who has been trained to keep people alive—to shift from aggressively treating a disease to accepting the reality that the patient likely will die.

In the best of all possible worlds, once your doctor can see that there is nothing medicine can do to keep you from dying, they would honestly and kindly deliver that information to you and discuss next steps. They would let you know what to expect as far as the progression of your disease and how to access hospice care.

Many doctors are ready and willing to discuss hospice care; others, unfortunately, are not. It's important to acknowledge that your doctors may not deliver information in the most straightforward way. Pay attention. Hear what your doctor is saying. If you're unsure, ask them to clarify.

Let's say that you've been battling an aggressive cancer. You might hear your oncologist say something that sounds like this: "We've done this treatment. We've tried that treatment. And right now, there's nothing more we can do." They may not be using the word *death* or *dying*, but that is likely what they are saying.

You also might hear something like this: "There's this other option, but you're too weak to receive it right now." It hurts my heart when a patient says to me, "My doctor said I'm too weak to stay on chemo, so we're going to go on hospice while I wait a few weeks to get stronger. Then I'll come off hospice and get back on chemo." More often than not, the oncologist knows that this patient is within weeks of death. Instead of being clear, the doctor has hedged around the hard conversation by making it about the patient's "strength."

I'll share with you the advice I'd give my own family members: If your oncologist says, "Let's see if we can get you stronger and go back on chemotherapy in a few weeks," consider beginning hospice. That's your signal. And guess what? If you do get stronger in three weeks, or eight weeks, then you *can* come off hospice and return to chemo. If treatments are no longer curing or controlling your disease, it's time to go on hospice.

In the absence of a transparent conversation with your doctor, you have to use your own judgment. If it is you who is dying, ask yourself: How comfortable am I? How functional am I? If it's your loved one, watch them and talk to them. Are they suffering? Are they struggling to take basic care of themselves?

At the end of the day, you have control. It's your decision, and clearer information about your disease and prognosis will help you make the best decision. If you don't know if it's the right time, I always say, "When in doubt, check it out." If you're curious about hospice, just check it out and see what you learn. You don't need a health-care professional to give you permission.

If treatments are no longer curing or controlling your disease, it's time to go on hospice.

How Do I Find a Hospice-Care Provider?

If you've made the decision to go on hospice, you'll need to choose a provider. Your doctor will give you a referral and you'll have a consultation, most likely in your home. Here's what I need you to know: you *do not* have to go with the first company you speak to. If you click with them right away, great! Sometimes the choice is that easy. At other times, it isn't. You may need time to consult with your family. Take that extra time. There are no obligations during your first visit.

If you do take additional time or want to interview other providers, you may need to request another referral from your doctor. You have a right to ask for that. That may mean some more work, but it also may mean the difference between living out the rest of your life the way you want or compromising. It's all your choice.

When looking for a hospice-care provider, word of mouth is always a good bet. Did your neighbor have a good experience caring for her dad in her home? Is there someone whom a colleague would recommend? Check in with those near you who've received hospice care.

You also can visit Medicare's website to look for a local provider. At the time of this writing, you can search for hospice-care providers in your area at medicare.gov/care-compare.

Who Is on a Hospice Team?

When you're receiving hospice care, the people you'll see most often are your hospice nurse and your hospice home health aide, but there is actually an entire team of professionals available to you, listed below. I encourage you to utilize all of your team members and get as much help as you can during this time. This is an all-hands-on-deck time. Your hospice team is here for you;

they want to provide support and help in whatever way they can. Let them.

Hospice Doctor

You'll likely see the hospice agency's nurse more often than you'll see your doctor, but the doctor is the one supervising your care, prescribing your medication, and making top-level decisions. A hospice doctor has the same kind of training and experience you'd expect from any other physician; they just happen to specialize in hospice care.

Hospice Nurse

This is me. Your hospice nurse is the face of hospice for you and works closely with your doctor to provide care—in fact, you can think of them as the doctor's eyes and ears. In addition to doing a full physical assessment each visit, they manage medications, symptoms, and any other issues that arise. They also can answer questions from you and your caregivers about your specific disease, the process of dying, and the ins and outs of hospice care. You'll see this person a lot. (It's good to note that usually one nurse will be your case manager, but you may have other nurses visit if it's the weekend, your nurse is on call or off sick, etc.)

Hospice Social Worker

The hospice company's social worker can help you navigate various social or personal challenges you may be facing. They also can help fill out forms applying for financial aid or other programs in your city or state that might be beneficial for you. If you have concerns about your safety, relationships, care, or anything else, ask to speak to your social worker.

Hospice Chaplain

In my experience, hospice chaplains are some of the best people you'll ever meet, but their visits are the ones patients decline to receive most often. Whether you're a person of faith or not, I would highly recommend allowing the chaplain to visit. They can help with existential questions, emotional support, and of course spiritual support if you want it. They can pray with you or just talk with you, whatever is best for you and your family.

Home Health Aide

Your hospice agency can provide you with a home health aide to assist your primary caregivers. The aide helps with dressing, changing, bathing, and other everyday tasks. Home health aides are amazing. They work together with nurses as a team, and you'll be seeing a lot of both.

Volunteers

Lots of people volunteer with hospice. Volunteers may call patients to check if they need medication refills or other supplies, or they may visit in person. Face-to-face visits can be for comfort and companionship—for example, to read to a person—or they can be for more practical tasks like shopping for groceries or helping clean up around the house.

Bereavement Specialist

After the person receiving hospice care dies, hospice agencies offer counseling, group sessions, and other resources for family members and loved ones for up to a year. The bereavement specialist coordinates these services. Please be sure to utilize these resources.

Do Hospice Patients Still Need Caregivers at Home?

Some people mistakenly assume that once they're on hospice, they no longer need any other caregivers. Although your hospice provider likely will be *available* twenty-four hours a day to answer your questions and even send a nurse if necessary, that's very different from providing around-the-clock care in your home. That means you *will* need additional help. Of course, you can hire a home health aide or other professional caregiver, but most likely the primary caregivers will be family, friends, or others who love the hospice patient. They'll be the ones providing meals, changing clothes, giving baths, and dispensing medications.

The lack of a caregiver at home is one of the biggest problems we see in hospice. This happens most often if someone doesn't have family members close by, or if family members work long hours. This is a common occurrence, and unfortunately, in our dysfunctional health-care system, there isn't always an easy answer. The hospice social worker can help you find caregivers (you'll have to pay out of pocket for these) or try to place the patient in a skilled nursing facility or hospice home, but that isn't always possible.

Because this can all feel like a lot, let me strongly advise you to *accept help that is offered*. I'm independent, too, and I know that I'll struggle with that if I end up on hospice care. I understand how difficult this can be. We want to do everything ourselves. We don't want to be a burden. But as I've spent time in countless homes with those who are dying, I've seen such beautiful acts of love and care that are mutually beneficial. Don't refuse help. Let other family members and friends step in to care for you. It can be a gift to you both.

Death Doulas

Many people who give birth choose to have a doula—someone who isn't a medical expert but is professionally trained to guide and support them during pregnancy and labor. A doula can offer tips, insights, and strategies to help someone through this new, foreign experience. There is now a growing movement of end-of-life doulas as well. They are trained to help the dying person and their family navigate the entire dying process. They are not medical caregivers, but they can supplement hospice care (and can be brought into the process much earlier than hospice workers). Death doulas can be of service in many ways—physical, emotional, and spiritual. They can help relieve exhausted caregivers or assist with financial planning and funeral preparations. More holistically, they can help with grief by coaching a family and the dying loved one through the natural death process. I have a lot of respect for this growing movement in the area of natural death, and I encourage you to do some more research on your own to learn about these wonderful caregivers.

Be Your Own Advocate

Technically, it is a patient's doctor who will eventually say that they are ready for hospice, but I strongly encourage patients, family members of patients, and other loved ones to be educated advocates. This may sound like I'm asking you to advocate for *death*, but what I'm really encouraging you to do is to advocate for *life*. When you're thoughtful and intentional about what the end of life might look like for you or your loved one, you are preparing not just to die well but also to live well.

So what's an educated advocate? Two things: First, you're educated. You've researched your disease, and you know what the symptoms are, what its progress is likely to be, and what kind of specific care you may need. Second, you advocate. You stand up for yourself, for your loved ones, and for a peaceful and comfortable death.

If your doctor doesn't bring up hospice care, you can bring it up yourself. When you do, notice the doctor's response. Are they comfortable discussing hospice care? Do they seem resistant? Are they quick to dismiss you, saying, "We're not there yet"? Many doctors are comfortable and well versed in the ins and outs of hospice care; others are not. If your doctor isn't, then you need to be. Again, be an educated advocate. And remember, when in doubt, check it out. You can call a hospice company yourself and ask questions, even without a doctor's referral.

Questions to Ask
before Signing Up for Hospice

Here are a few questions to ask hospice companies before signing up, along with the answers you ideally want to hear:

Q: How many patients does each nurse have on their caseload?

A: Twelve to fifteen (usually); if it's greater than fifteen, the nurse may have too many patients to care for them all effectively.

Q: What types of methods do you use to manage pain?

A: Examples include oral medications, liquid medications, continuous ambulatory delivery device (CADD) pumps, and pain patches.

Q: What kinds of care do you offer if symptoms can't be managed?

A: Continuous-care nursing or inpatient hospice care.

And remember, if you're dissatisfied with the care your hospice company is providing, you can always switch to another one.

Choose What's Right for You

I love hospice. In my years as a hospice nurse, I've seen dying people and their loved ones well served by the care that we offer. But I would never push someone who didn't need or want it toward hospice care. My goal is to promote peaceful death. If you're getting that without hospice? Wonderful! I recognize that it may *not* be right for everyone. Even if a person is eligible, it still might not be right for them. A person may meet the requirements, but if they're still living independently and comfortably and don't yet need help with symptom management, then that person should do what brings them the most comfort during their end-of-life journey.

On the other hand, I may see a patient who is strongly opposed to receiving hospice care and has only accepted my visit to appease loved ones. Or if the patient isn't alert during my visit, it may be that the family is resistant to hospice. Maybe this patient or their family doesn't yet realize how very sick they are or hasn't been given a clear explanation of their condition. When this is the case, I'll take the time to educate them about their disease and what's happening to them. I'll let them know what I've seen in my experience with similar patients, and I'll tell them what I'm noticing about them. I won't leave before I'm sure that everyone involved has a good grasp of the disease and its likely progression.

In the end, though, every situation is different. I hope that you'll gather as much information as you can. Learn about your disease. Talk to your doctor. Consult with as many hospice companies as you need to become comfortable. Educate yourself and your loved ones. Do whatever it takes so that you have everything you need when the time comes to make the very best decision for *you*.

Chapter 4

Clean, Safe, and Comfortable

A s I've now discussed at length, there's a big difference between medical care with the goal of curing, healing, or saving the life of an otherwise healthy patient and medical care with the goal of supporting a patient on their end-of-life journey. When we are talking about the latter, hospice care's main goal is to manage your symptoms at home, so you truly *live* the rest of your life. We are here to support you and your family so you can carry out the things you've been wanting to do. In the end, hospice care can boil down to these three questions:

1. Is the person clean?

2. Is the person safe?

3. Is the person comfortable?

Truly, I believe that asking these three questions can be a game changer for hospice patients and caregivers. When you can answer these three questions in the affirmative, you can give yourself permission to let go of a lot of other things.

If a person is no longer able to care for themselves, the responsibility of keeping them clean, safe, and comfortable falls to the caregivers. What can be a bit tricky, though, is when a person who's always been independent, and still is mostly independent, *refuses* care. This is why "clean, safe, and comfortable" can be so useful. Determining whether a loved one is clean, safe, and comfortable helps a caregiver discern when to push and when to let something go.

Determining whether a loved one is clean, safe, and comfortable helps a caregiver discern when to push and when to let something go.

When we ask whether someone is clean, safe, and comfortable, it's just another way of letting their bodies guide them—and guide their caregivers. So one day the person on hospice might feel like getting up and baking cookies. The next day, the same person might choose to spend the day in bed. A lot of families begin to worry when their loved ones begin sleeping for long stretches at a time. They may fear that the additional slumber is cutting into nutrition or socializing or exercising. I understand.

Although it can feel a little counterintuitive to everything we know about the well-being of people who are physically healthy, I encourage family members to allow the person who is sick to decide how much they want to sleep, how much they want to move their body, and how much they want to eat. This isn't the time for the dying person to keep up with a workout routine, watch what they eat, or kick every bad habit in their lives. This is the time for the person who is sick to make their own choices about their body, as they're able, while remaining clean, safe, and comfortable.

How to Tell If Someone Is Clean, Safe, and Comfortable

We can visually observe whether someone is clean and safe, but some people don't have the ability to tell us verbally that they're comfortable. When you're with a dying person who is unresponsive or no longer able to communicate effectively, it's natural to be concerned that they might be in pain and just can't tell you.

If that's you, I want to relieve you of that fear. People who are losing their abilities—even their ability to communicate verbally—still can effectively communicate when they're uncomfortable or in distress. This is another incredible way that our bodies were built to die. Think about this. Infants communicate their discomfort all the time, despite having zero language skills. When a person who is nonverbal or actively dying is wet, agitated, in pain, or otherwise uncomfortable, they will find ways to let you know. Like an infant, they may not be using language, but there are other signs to look for, even if they're unconscious:

- They may seem agitated or exhibit restlessness.

- They may wince in pain or distress.

- They may furrow their brow.

- Their body might tighten up or show sudden stiffness.

- They may be touching a body part that hurts.

- When touched, they may act guarded, shifting to protect an area.

These are reliable signals that alert us that a body may be in pain. When we notice them, we can respond by looking for the most obvious reasons it might be happening, which might include the following:

- Is the person wet or soiled?

- Is the person constipated?

- Do they have any wounds?

- Are there signs of any other injury?

- Does their mouth need to be moistened?

I know you can feel helpless when your loved one doesn't communicate the way they used to. But if you remain attentive to these other signs, you still can offer the care they need. And remember, if you have questions or concerns, you can always talk to your hospice nurse. Nurses and physicians are professionally trained to use several nonverbal pain scales to determine a patient's level of pain or discomfort.

Managing Pain

One of the biggest myths about dying is that death in and of itself is painful. Well, I have good news for you: this is not true. The disease a person is dying from can cause pain, but actual death itself is not painful. Our bodies are built to be born, and they're built to die. If someone was to live to be a hundred years old and die naturally of old age without any terminal illness, they most likely would not have any pain at death. However, because most people die from specific diseases, and because the symptoms of those diseases can be painful, many people equate death with pain. Hospice can manage those symptoms for you and help you have a peaceful death. The task of the entire care team is to figure out the best ways to manage the specific pain a person may be feeling, which varies by disease.

Hospice nurses are experts at managing pain. We have long-acting pain medicine. We have short-acting pain medicine. We have pain pills, suppositories, injections, CADD pumps, and many other forms of pain medicine delivery. If you're on hospice and your pain isn't managed, you need to talk to somebody. Like, *now*. You do not have to die in pain.

You do not have to die in pain.

Now, if the dying person isn't uncomfortable, there may be no need to administer pain medication. However, if the person is experiencing pain, we can be as aggressive as we need to be in managing it. Your hospice nurse will *never* administer pain medication without justification. We are not here to just "drug you up"! Be an advocate for yourself or your loved one, and allow us to help you.

The Benefits of Morphine

The most common pain medication at the end of life is liquid morphine, which can help a person with pain and shortness of breath (often called "air hunger"). I find that many people have concerns about administering morphine, and I want to put some of those fears to rest.

Some people mistakenly may believe that morphine "kills" people, or at least hastens their death. One reason people think this is that morphine slows breathing. This is true, but the amount of morphine we administer to patients on hospice is so minimal that breathing will not slow to the point of respiratory arrest. Research published in the journal *Cancer* demonstrates that hospice patients who receive morphine die more peacefully, but they do not die *sooner* than those who don't receive morphine. People on hospice are dying; they will die whether we give morphine or not.

Typically, we offer a very minimal amount of liquid morphine underneath the tongue, where it's easily absorbed through the gum tissue. This small dose relaxes the diaphragm and the central nervous system, which helps a person who feels like they can't get a good or deep breath breathe more comfortably.

Trust me when I assure you that morphine helps people who are dying; it doesn't hurt them. If someone is suffering as they die, morphine helps control and manage their pain so they can die more peacefully.

Bradyn, just nineteen years old, was on hospice care for advanced-stage cancer. Before being on hospice, he'd been on low-dose pain meds that never helped him control the pain he had been experiencing as a result of his cancer.

He would say, "All I could do was lie in bed and do nothing. Or sleep."

Once Bradyn came on hospice, it was our recommendation that he begin using morphine as a palliative aid. Like a lot of us, he was afraid. The word *morphine* made him think of recreational drug users, criminals, and addiction. He'd basically been told his whole life that morphine was bad. From parents to teachers to TV, morphine is regularly depicted as being the cause of a lot of trouble and something to be avoided at all costs.

Here's the thing, though: when ordered and monitored by a qualified medical professional and used by patients who have received a terminal diagnosis, morphine is not only perfectly safe, it's also practically a miracle drug. In my experience, nothing works better to relieve pain in the terminally ill, and when you reduce pain, you reduce suffering.

After we discussed it with him and his family, Bradyn did allow us to administer him morphine. He had an immediate improvement in his quality of life. In Bradyn's words, "Once hospice helped me get my pain under control, I was able to start doing things I couldn't do before. I had energy to get up and walk around. I played video games with my little brother. I know that doesn't sound like much, but it's something I couldn't do before. Hospice has changed my life from feeling like I'm dying to feeling like I'm living again."

The Comfort Kit

One of the resources we provide to people on hospice is a comfort kit containing several medications, including morphine or another opioid, antianxiety meds, antiemetics for nausea, bronchodilators, and over-the-counter pain and constipation relievers. A person doesn't have to use them if they're not needed, but they're readily available in case of emergency. This can be incredibly useful when your hospice nurse isn't present (for example, in the middle of the night) or when for some reason a regular pain reliever isn't working. As always, consult your hospice team with any questions or concerns.

Here's what's in the comfort kit (may vary slightly from hospice to hospice):

1. Morphine, used for pain and shortness of breath

2. Lorazepam, used for anxiety, agitation, and restlessness

3. Hyoscyamine, used to dry up excess secretions that cause the "death rattle"

4. Zofran, used for nausea and vomiting, if needed (although most people don't have nausea and vomiting at the end of life)

5. Tylenol suppository, used for end-of-life fevers

6. Bisacodyl suppository, used for constipation

7. Bisacodyl pill, used for constipation

8. Haldol, used for agitation

Note that because it can be difficult for patients to swallow at the end of life, we don't use pills or liquids that need to be swallowed. The meds in the comfort kit are almost all taken either rectally (as a suppository) or sublingually (absorbed through the gum tissue under the tongue, with no swallowing necessary).

The Sedation Myth

Many people think that when a person goes on hospice care, we sedate them until they die. We do not. Our goal is to give the dying person a better *life* in addition to a better death. We would never simply "knock someone out" and be done with it.

I think this misconception arises when people see someone they know come on hospice *too late*. They might have seen someone with previously unmanaged symptoms who was in a lot of distress before they even came to us. In these cases, we *are* aggressive with our treatments because the person may have been in extreme pain or discomfort for some time, and we need to get them comfortable quickly. To an outsider, these cases may look like, "You just sedated them and then they died." But that's not what happened. In reality, this person unfortunately would have died whether we gave them medication or not, but in giving medication, we allowed them to die peacefully.

Our Bodies Are Built to Die

After years as a hospice nurse, I can share this strange but true fact: *our bodies are biologically built to die*. Again, think about infants. Our bodies are made to survive birth and to receive what they need in infancy. For example, babies are born with a sucking reflex, and this instinct equips them to receive the nourishment they need to thrive. Similarly, our bodies, if left alone during the dying process (with nothing being forced on them), usually will help us die a peaceful death. This means that at the end of life, many natural impulses that healthy people need to survive begin to shut down when they are no longer needed.

The most important way this phenomenon manifests is this: when dying a natural death, your body instinctively shuts down the mechanism that makes you feel hungry and thirsty. How miraculous is that? As your body has less and less need for food and water, sensations of hunger and thirst disappear. This makes perfect sense because a naturally dying body loses the ability to swallow, so eating and drinking become more difficult. These natural functions are the body's way of taking care of the person who is dying.

These changes can be distressing, especially for caregivers

who begin to notice that their loved one is refusing food and water. But this refusal not only is normal, it's to be expected! This person isn't dying because they're not eating and drinking; rather, they're not eating and drinking because they're dying. Because our bodies know how to die, the less we mess with the body's natural dying process, the more peaceful the death will be.

This person isn't dying because they're not eating and drinking; rather, they're not eating and drinking because they're dying.

Against Forced Hydration

Not only do our bodies need less hydration during the dying process, but too much fluid actually can be harmful. I know this sounds counterintuitive. For most of our lives, we've been encouraged to stay hydrated. It's good for our brains. It aids digestion. It helps with headaches. It gives us more energy. It prevents kidney stones. Most of us can't imagine going without water and not suffering.

But the truth is, at the end of life, hydration actually causes more problems than it solves. People at the end of life *should* be dehydrated. When a person is naturally dehydrated at the end of life, the body releases endorphins that make the person more comfortable. These natural painkillers are the body's way of taking care of the person who is dying.

To be clear, I'm not saying that a caregiver should ever deny fluids to a patient who's expressing that they're thirsty. If they're thirsty, please give them a drink. If they're no longer able to swallow, you can offer them some water or juice on a sponge, or if they can swallow a bit without choking, you can offer a Popsicle or ice cream. But when a dying person starts refusing water, inevitably, the family will ask if we should start intravenous (IV) fluids. That means delivering fluids into the bloodstream through an IV catheter that's inserted into a vein in the patient's arm, as is standard practice in a hospital.

The answer is no.

When I was an ICU nurse, I wouldn't have believed what I'm saying today. (And if you're a nurse who hasn't worked hospice, you might never be exposed to this information.) In the ICU, this kind of intravenous hydration is how we keep people alive. When a hospital patient *isn't* in the final stages of dying and they need IV hydration, ten times out of ten they'll receive it.

But at the end of life, the body is not working as it once did, and it simply doesn't have a way to process all that IV fluid. The heart is no longer pumping as efficiently as it used to, and the extra hydration just doesn't stay in the vascular system. It seeps out, causing ascites (swelling of the abdomen) or edema (swelling of the limbs and extremities). Eventually, it backs up into the lungs, causing respiratory distress, which is one of the worst sensations we as humans can have. If someone is having enough respiratory distress, they may have to be intubated, meaning a tube will be inserted through their mouth and down into their lungs so a machine can breathe for them. In the ICU, for a patient who is expected to live, this makes sense. The breathing machine will breathe for them until they get better and can be taken off the machine. But in hospice, when end of life is certain and the patient is terminal, the goal becomes more comfort focused, and a breathing machine is not something we could or should do. All of this is to say: the side effects of forced hydration are not peaceful and usually cause more harm to our loved one on hospice.

Oral Care at the End of Life

Oral care at the end of life is something you can provide to comfort and support your loved one who can no longer swallow. To moisten their mouth, you have a few options:

- Ice chips
- Sponge with cold water
- Washcloth with cold water

Remember to moisten the person's tongue and inner mouth as well as their lips.

I visited with Jean as her family switched her from palliative care to hospice care. Due to a large tumor in her stomach, Jean was no longer able to eat and had been on IV hydration and nutrition for several months. As a result, her abdomen and legs were swollen, causing her a lot of discomfort and shortness of breath. Her doctor had ordered the insertion of a small tube called a PleurX drain into her abdomen to drain the fluid. Although it relieved the problem in the short term, it wasn't a fix-all solution.

I wanted to make sure Jean and her husband understood what was happening in her body.

"IV fluids and nutrition are, technically, keeping you alive," I explained. "But the fluid is not staying in your vascular system. It's seeping out. All the hydration you're receiving is causing the swelling and shortness of breath. It may be delaying your death, but it's also making your life harder than it needs to be."

I knew that was a lot to process, so I paused to leave some space for them to make sense of what I'd said.

"So," Jean's husband asked cautiously, "what's the alternative?"

"Well," I answered gently, "you could choose to stop the hydration, and you'd feel more comfortable. You could possibly die quicker, but you'd also die more peacefully."

In the end, Jean stopped her IV nutrition. Her swelling decreased, and so did her pain and shortness of breath. During visits she would say to me, "I finally feel better." She lived for about two more weeks, and during those two weeks, she had fewer symptoms and was able to more fully enjoy her last few good days with her family.

It can be hard for caregivers and professionals to make the mental shift from "hydration is good" to "hydration is bad." But the fact of the matter is that the person who is naturally dehydrated will be more comfortable, while the person who is being artificially hydrated will experience more discomfort and suffering. If you want your loved one to have the opportunity for a peaceful, natural, beautiful death, let them be dehydrated at the very end. The body knows how to die. Let it.

The Most Important Thing

In the end, the most important thing for anxious loved ones to remember are the three questions we started the chapter with: Is my person clean? Is my person safe? Is my person comfortable? Hospice is available to make sure the answer to all three questions is yes.

We're here to support you and your loved ones as your body dies. You don't have to live with unmanaged symptoms. Hospice can help.

Chapter 5

What the Dying Process Looks Like

In this chapter, we'll take a closer look at what the process of dying usually looks like. We'll start with the big picture, reviewing the signs you might see beginning about six months from death, and then go over what to expect during the final days and hours. Wherever you might be in your journey toward death, be gentle with yourself. If you're beating yourself up for something like not exercising or sleeping too much, you need to let yourself off the hook. This isn't the time for rigorous self-improvement. Be kind to yourself.

I know that not everyone has witnessed a natural death, one that's the result of natural causes such as age or disease rather than an accident or violence. If you've chosen to die a natural death on hospice, you won't receive interventions to extend your life. You won't get CT scans, PET scans, or chemotherapy. You won't undergo radiation unless it's for a palliative reason, such as to keep you comfortable. You won't be admitted to the hospital. (If you choose to return to the hospital and resume medical interventions for a disease, then you'll be taken off hospice care.)

That doesn't mean you won't get any medical care. Hospice can and will treat many issues, focusing on how you feel and what we can do to help. We still can treat infections, give antibiotics, treat wounds, and so on. If it will help manage symptoms and keep you comfortable, and Medicare allows it, we will do it.

But as amazing as all that is, I want you to know that you actually already have a guide on your journey toward death. It is *your body*.

Your body was built for death, and it knows how to die. Let your body be your guide. No one, no matter how well trained or how brilliant, can know what it feels like to be inside your body. No one else knows how you feel. Only you do.

When your body is your guide, you listen to what it's telling you. When you pay attention to your body, you eat when you're hungry and drink when you're thirsty. You sleep when you're tired and take pain medications when you're in pain. Accept your body where it is, and trust that it knows how to take care of you. Because it does.

"How Long Do I Have?"

I can answer a lot of the questions my patients and their families ask, but there are some that I can't. Probably the most frequent question I get from patients—and the one that's the most difficult to answer, at least precisely—is, "How long do I have?"

I love this question because it means they want to know the

facts about their condition. As with the rest of the dying process, the more information you have, the more power you have in deciding how you want to live before you die. I think a lot of people believe doctors and nurses are trying to hide something when they hesitate to answer this question, that maybe they're just trying to appease the dying person and not deliver bad news. That's usually not the case. Often, it's just too difficult to know how long someone has left to live, and so there really is no answer to give.

If I could give a precise answer to this question, I'd do it. I love living in the black and white as much as anyone else. It feels safe. Unfortunately, it's a really difficult question to answer because so much can happen in the last six months of life, and quickly. Also, everyone's death is an individual experience. Your death won't necessarily look like somebody else's. People are simply different. In the same way that your *life* may have looked nothing like the life of someone with a similar background to yours, your *death* won't look like theirs either. It's especially tough to know how long someone has left when a death is expected to be at least three to six months out. As a death gets closer, it becomes a little easier to estimate, but there's still a lot of gray area, a lot of unknown.

That said, if you have received a terminal diagnosis—meaning you've been told you're going to die—and have chosen to die a natural death on hospice, you can expect to see a few common changes start to happen. If you're not used to listening to your body or if you're unfamiliar with natural death, here are some things you or your loved one may experience at the beginning of the process:

- **Social withdrawal:** You'll become more interested in being alone than being with people. You'll likely spend a lot more time in your room and sleep a lot more. That's okay.

- **Functional decline:** First, it may become more difficult for you to leave the house. Then it may become more difficult for you to leave the room. Finally, it may become difficult for you to leave the bed. Eventually you'll need total care.

- **Decrease in appetite:** As your body begins to shut down, you'll naturally become less interested in food and water. That's okay.

- **Increase in sleep:** You'll begin to sleep more. You may notice you're asleep more than you're awake. That's okay.

- **Mental status decline:** Mental status doesn't change for everyone, but many people experience intermittent confusion and disorientation, especially when first waking up or in the evening. Mental status changes can depend on specific disease processes.

The Last Six Months of Life

As I mentioned, it's impossible to know exactly what a given person's last six months will look like, but we can know *something* about how the journey toward death will unfold by looking at the person's diagnosis. Many diseases unfold in relatively pre-dictable patterns.

When a disease progresses at a consistent pace, for example, we call it a "downward slope," and we expect the person to de-cline steadily and predictably. As time passes, the person will become progressively less able to live the way they once did. End-stage cancer is usually like this.

Other diseases progress more like a "staircase": during a lon-ger period of time, with plateaus that precede various declines. In these cases, someone may be living fairly well with their dis-ease and then a sudden incident occurs that causes a decline. They may have a fall or develop an infection, for example, and quickly slide down to another plateau, where again they will live fairly consistently until the next incident, and so on, until death. Some of the chronic terminal illnesses we expect to show this staircase pattern include ALS, Parkinson's, COPD, and conges-tive heart failure.

A frustrating consequence of the staircase-type progression is that during the plateau stages of the disease, the dying person might no longer qualify for hospice care. It's not necessarily be-cause the person is improving, but rather because they may simply no longer meet all the criteria for hospice. Ultimately, when they take that next step down, they will become eligible once more.

Following is a typical timeline seen in the natural dying pro-cess. During the last six months, there will be a gradual decline until death. The farther out you are, the more intermittent and infrequent the signs are. You may see only slight changes in behavior at first, but the closer you get to the end, the more acute and regular they'll become.

Six to three months from death

- Slightly increased sleepiness

- Social withdrawal

- Eating and drinking less

Three months to one month from death

- Decreasing food and water intake

- Slow decline in physical function, needing help with tasks like food prep, showering, getting to the bathroom, and other self-care

- Continuous lethargy

- Sleeping a lot more than normal

- Gradual mental decline, including some intermittent disorientation or confusion

- Possibly becoming homebound or bedridden

One month from death

- Minimal food and water intake

- More and more acute physical and mental decline

- "Visioning," or seeing dead loved ones (See chapter 6 for more information on this phenomenon.)

- In and out of consciousness, likely eventually unconscious

Days and hours from death (actively dying)

- Little consciousness

- Unresponsive, or mostly unresponsive

- Likely not eating and drinking at all

- Bedridden and incontinent

- Changes in breathing, skin color, and temperature

- Noisy breath

- Possible terminal lucidity, or "rallying" (See chapter 6 for more on this.)

The Actively Dying Phase

In the final days and hours of a person's life, they enter what is called the "actively dying" phase. It's here that you're going to see the biggest changes in a dying person's body and behavior.

One of the most distressing things I hear from my followers on social media is that they believe they saw their loved ones *suf-*

fer at the end of life. I never want to negate anyone's experience, because I wasn't there and I'm not them, but in general, what these people are describing as suffering is simply what actively dying looks like. It's just that no one had told them that what they were seeing was normal or why it was happening.

Because we talk about death so little in our society, most people don't know what they're seeing when a person is actively dying. If I wasn't a hospice nurse who sees it all the time, I would think it's scary, too. So I want you to know what's happening as the human body shuts down. I want you to know what kind of breathing to expect. What kinds of sights and sounds to expect. What kind of behavior to expect. Most importantly, I want you to know that during a natural death, although the actively dying phase may look unusual, scary, or even traumatic, everything that's happening is normal. The actively dying person is *not* suffering.

So what does actively dying look like? Let's break it down in detail.

The actively dying person is not *suffering.*

Changes in Sleeping, Eating, and Speaking

Sleeping is a huge part of the dying process. It's typical for a person who's dying to sleep more than eighteen hours a day, and sometimes as much as twenty-four hours a day. At the end of life, the body's calcium levels rise. This causes sleepiness and is one of the body's built-in mechanisms to help us die. The dying person will start to sleep more and more, until finally, at the very end of life, they will be entirely unconscious. In addition, when someone is actively dying, they will be unresponsive, even to tactile stimulation. Although these signals would be troubling to see in a person who's healthy, they are absolutely to be expected in a person who's dying.

The person who's dying also won't be eating or drinking. When a person stops taking in food and liquid, the body goes into a metabolic state called "ketosis." (If that word looks familiar, it's probably because it is the same state people try to achieve with the keto diet. It's sort of an extreme metabolism that the body can enter into for many reasons, not just death.) In the later phases of ketosis, the nervous system is dulled. As a result, the person who's not eating or drinking isn't feeling pain, thirst, or hunger. They may even feel a sense of euphoria.

Additionally, the dying person likely won't be speaking at the end. Despite what we see in the movies, people usually don't deliver an inspiring monologue moments before death. Many people don't realize that it takes a lot of energy to speak. Air has to be pushed out of the lungs and over the vocal cords. When someone is close to death, their diaphragm is weak. They don't have the energy to get that air through their vocal cords to use their voice normally. When the person *is* still able to speak, the voice may sound different from how it usually sounds. It may be raspy and quiet. Eventually, however, the person at the end of life will stop speaking altogether.

Nonverbal Pain Scales

When a person is unconscious, we can determine whether they're in pain or not by using nonverbal pain scales and by watching the person's body language.

Changes in Breathing

It's very normal for the actively dying person's breathing patterns to change. One common pattern is called "fish out of water" breathing and looks like short, rapid, shallow breaths. Another is Cheyne-Stokes breathing, which is described as deep, rapid breaths followed by a long pause.

When witnessing such changes in breathing, many people think their loved one is in distress. Although this change in the pace and sound of breath can be disturbing, it's not uncomfortable for the person who is dying. It's just their body's way of shutting down. Despite the unfamiliar rhythm, the person who's having a change in breathing is *not* panicking. We know that because, when we look at them, even when their breathing is irregular, they appear relaxed.

Now, if the person does show us, via nonverbal cues, that they're particularly uncomfortable, we'll medicate them. But those changes in breathing at the end of life are a very normal part of the process.

Changes in Skin Color and Temperature

During the last few days or hours of a person's life, we expect to see some changes in a person's skin color. This is called "mottling." We see mottling when the heart is no longer able to pump blood effectively. As blood pressure drops, blood flow slows, and the dying person's extremities can begin to feel cold to the touch, too. We may see mottling first in the feet and hands, possibly the knees or the tip of the nose. On pale skin, the extremities may turn a little purplish, bluish, or reddish, or they may appear marbled. The discoloration can be solid or patchy. On darker skin, mottling can be more difficult to identify, but circulatory changes still will result in cooler extremities. None of this is painful to the dying person. It's just another signal that the body is in the process of shutting down.

Terminal Secretions, or the "Death Rattle"

When a person is actively dying, you may hear a wet rasping or gurgling sound with every breath. This sound has been nicknamed the "death rattle," and it's probably the symptom that causes families the most distress. People who hear it usually fear that their loved one is drowning in fluid bubbling up from their lungs. If you've heard this sound and this was your first reaction, you're not alone. I've been with countless families who have been seriously disturbed by it. But like other biological changes during the actively dying phase, the death rattle is nothing to fear.

Here is why that sound is happening: We produce saliva all the time. When we're healthy, our brains signal us to swallow it. When we're dying, that mechanism shuts down, and we no longer can physically swallow. The saliva then builds up in the mouth, making the breath sound "wet." The person who's dying is likely breathing with their mouth open because their muscles are relaxed. This increases airflow, and all of that air then passes over the saliva, creating a rattling or gurgling sound. In addition to hearing a sound, you also may see fluid in the mouth and throat.

Sometimes family members want to get rid of the terminal secretions, and in the ICU we're taught to be aggressive about suctioning out secretions. But that's not necessarily best for the person who's dying. In fact, it can be harmful. Suctioning out the saliva causes the body to produce even more. So doing this might actually end up creating *more* noise, not less, and might cause additional problems that would then need to be addressed. There are medications we can give to dry the secretions and lessen the sound, however. Repositioning or turning the person can help as well.

I can't emphasize enough that the body knows what it's doing during death, just like it does at birth. A newborn baby can make all sorts of concerning noises, but when it's really in trouble, you know it. *Because it will tell you.* It cries or winces or gives some other indication that it is in pain. It's exactly the same with the dying. The death rattle is not an indication of suffering. The dying person will show signs of true distress if there is something really wrong.

Open Eyes and Mouth

When a person is actively dying, their eyes and mouth likely will be open. In regular, everyday life, we're used to seeing our loved ones with their eyes open. During death, however, people get concerned because the dying person's eyes might be open but they're not making eye contact, or just one eye is open or partially open. This happens because it takes a lot of muscles to blink our eyes or keep them shut. During the actively dying phase, those muscles are relaxed and no longer working unconsciously so the eyes stay open or partially open.

Family members are often also bothered when they see a dying person's mouth hanging open. The person's tongue may even be sticking out. Again, this is simply a sign that the person's muscles are very relaxed. It's almost like the body knows that those muscles are no longer needed, and it gives them a break. The brain basically stops communicating with those muscles.

I think the open eyes and mouth can be troubling because so often in our everyday lives, we don't even think about these functions. We're likely not even aware that muscles are required to close our eyelids or keep our mouths shut. But it's the way the body works. A mouth hanging open at the end of life and eyes that are open but not focused are entirely normal parts of the dying process. It simply means the body is relaxed.

Changes in Body Temperature

At the end of life, we lose the ability to control our core body temperature, and it may fluctuate. This can happen anywhere from a few days to a few hours before death. A person might spike a high fever, or they may get really, really cold. Again, this is totally normal and usually causes no discomfort. However, when it does seem uncomfortable for the dying person, there are interventions we can offer. If you're ever concerned, the first thing to do is call your hospice nurse. As you're learning, though, most of the time no interventions are necessary, and what you're seeing is the natural process of dying.

Maintaining a Comfortable Temperature

It's completely normal for your loved one's body temperature to change at the end of life, but if they seem uncomfortable, there are measures you can take.

If the person is hot:
- Set up portable fans.
- Provide cold compresses on the forehead, armpits, or inner elbows.
- Offer Tylenol in suppository form. (Ask your hospice team for details.)

If the person is cold:
- Provide warm blankets.
- Offer heating pads.

Fluid Release

Throughout our lives, we do our best to manage our bodily fluids. We diaper babies. We use tissues to dab away tears and catch our sneezes. We use deodorant and sweatbands to keep perspiration at bay. Women use pads to catch menstrual blood. As we age, we may even find ourselves back in diapers again.

At the end of life, it's reasonable to expect that feces, urine, tears, mucus, perspiration, and even blood will escape from our bodies. The types of fluid release you may see in your loved one around the time of death include the following:

- Urine from the bladder

- Stool from the bowels

- Fluid from the mouth and/or nose

- Tears from the eyes

- Foamy substances (white, brown, black, or bloody) escaping from the nose, mouth, and rectum

As with certain other end-of-life changes, this happens because of muscle relaxation. During life, many of the fluids in our bodies are unconsciously but actively being held in by muscles called sphincters. At the time of death, when we see a release of urine or stool, for example, it's because the body is *fully* relaxed. The bladder and the sphincters relax. The same holds true for all other orifices.

As a death and dying educator, I try to take the mystery out of a lot of what we see as people are dying. When we know what's happening, we can live better and die better. But I'm also careful not to try to tie it all up with a pretty bow. The reality is that some of it is just . . . *messy*. It is. Given a choice, we'd likely forego a lot of this mess. But it is what it is. What you're seeing—although it may not always be pleasant—is absolutely typical in death and dying and is not causing your loved one any discomfort.

Other Signs That the Body Is Shutting Down

Here are some other unfamiliar gestures or movements you may see or hear during the actively dying stage:

- **Teeth grinding:** Releasing energy through grinding or gritting the teeth is completely normal. It doesn't mean your loved one is in distress. When in doubt, always speak to your hospice team.

- **Growling:** Sometimes when we see teeth grinding, it can be paired with a noise that sounds like a growl. I know it can feel concerning for family members, but I've seen it often, and it's normal.

- **Tears:** The person who is dying may have teardrops rolling down their cheeks just as they die. This may be a physiological response of the body; because the dying person hasn't been blinking, the eyes are creating extra moisture for lubrication. I believe this is more of a biological response than an emotional one. In my experience, you don't need to worry that the person is upset.

- **Silent scream:** This is when the dying person opens their eyes and mouth wide and makes a face that looks like a silent scream. This can be creepy because we have associations with this look from horror films. Again, it's just relaxed muscles. There's no reason to assume that the person who makes this face is experiencing pain or fear.

This isn't a comprehensive list. You may experience some of these phenomena during the actively dying phase, or you may not. You may see unusual behavior that I haven't addressed. Whatever it is you witness, I want your takeaway to be this:

- The body knows how to die; what you're seeing is probably normal.

- The dying person likely isn't suffering.

- When in doubt, call your hospice nurse. That's what they're there for: to help you through this process and make your loved one's death as comfortable as possible.

Terminal Agitation

An elderly man who's in the process of actively dying is lying in bed. He's restless, kicking his legs around. Sometimes his legs will stretch out over the bed's safety bars and climb up the wall. He's stuffed a pillowcase in his shorts. His fingers are constantly picking at the bedsheets. These kinds of restless behaviors are normal, and we recognize them as possible signs of "terminal agitation." Someone else with terminal agitation might be trying continuously to get out of a chair or bed. They're constantly trying to go somewhere. They're usually disoriented, and there's no reasoning with this person.

Even though someone who is dying may be fidgety in these ways, the first thing we want to do is to make sure that they're not uncomfortable. If those behaviors are signaling that the person is in *distress*, we want to identify that and help manage it.

Nurses are trained to assess patients for nonverbal cues that tell us what they might be experiencing. When we identify these conditions, there are ways we can treat and help the person. When we're checking a patient for discomfort, we're looking to see if the person is communicating that they're experiencing any of the following:

1. Pain

2. Urine retention

3. Impacted bowels

If we don't identify any of those three things and aren't finding other evident signs of pain and discomfort, we can safely assume that the person is experiencing terminal agitation, or a restlessness that we sometimes see before death.

Several indicators may signal terminal agitation:

- Restlessness

- Appearing irritated or distressed

- Appearing uncomfortable

- Moving around continuously

- Fidgeting or pulling at things

- Attempting to get out of bed

When these things are happening, the person is generally disoriented. There's no use trying to reason with them or ask them to settle down. So if you're noticing these signs and would like to help your loved one relax, you may want to offer something that they find soothing. For some, it's music. For others, it's a quiet room with low stimulation. One woman seemed to be comforted when the lights were off and her family played an old movie at low volume. Another woman was soothed by a gentle hand massage. When one woman was tugging endlessly at her clothing, the family removed her clothing to decrease stimuli. You know your loved one and can experiment to offer them the most peaceful environment possible.

Typically, the person who is experiencing this terminal agitation isn't in distress that should worry us. But if they're at risk of harm in any way, then a hospice nurse can medicate them to help them calm down, rest, and stay safe. When the alternatives are either sleep or someone experiencing a disturbing amount of distress, sleep may be the kindest solution. Our main goal in serving the person who is dying is to keep them comfortable. Often, when the person wakes up after the medication wears off, they're less agitated.

When we've ruled out physical causes for a person's distress, we also can consider the possibility that they may be experiencing a more *existential* pain. We might naturally assume that no one *wants* to die, but the reality is that not everyone is resistant to the same degree. We may see extra resistance in someone who is young and wants to keep living, someone with unfinished business, or someone who is generally angsty, neurotic, anxious, or controlling.

When I witness someone who's extra resistant to letting go of life, I may ask their loved ones, "During his life, was he controlling? Stubborn? Independent?" And nine times out of ten, the family will burst out laughing. It actually can give the family a bit of relief because as they're seeing something they don't understand, they're often eager for answers. This answer—that the way we die often reflects the way we lived—makes sense to them. It's not a perfect answer, but for many it can be a helpful explanation.

How to Tell If a Dying Person Is Suffering

Families often wonder how we know their loved one isn't suffering. I like to describe a dying person like a baby. A baby who cannot communicate verbally that something is wrong will show us through their body language instead. They'll fuss. They'll cry. They'll be restless. A person who's dying will do the same thing. They'll be agitated. They'll moan. They'll furrow their brow. They'll physically show us. Really, it's pretty easy to tell a comfortable dying person from an uncomfortable one.

Another way hospice nurses can tell if a person is suffering is by using a nonverbal pain scale. This tool allows us to measure the degree of a patient's discomfort with great accuracy.

Lastly, we also record patients' vital signs. Body temperature, pulse rate, respiration rate, and blood pressure are measurements of critical bodily functions and can sometimes indicate if someone is in pain.

I don't put a lot of stock in vitals for hospice work, and I encourage family members not to worry about them too much either. Instead, be mindful of how the person who is dying tells you they're feeling, verbally or nonverbally.

If something's wrong, we'll treat it. For example, someone's oxygen level may look great when it's measured, but the person may still feel short of breath. We can treat that easily. On the other hand, someone's oxygen levels may look bad, but they feel fine. I'm good with that. It's all about how they feel and how they look.

Factors We Can't Control

I believe that we can be instrumental in choosing the type of death we'll have, yet there are some factors that we can't control:

- Age: Both the dying person and their loved ones are likely to be far more prepared to let go when the one in the bed is ninety-eight years old than when they're eighteen. And for relatively young people, under age fifty or so, it may be that only one part of their body is failing while the rest is still healthy and vibrant, which can make death more of a struggle.

- **Disease:** The type of disease a person is dying from can play a role in whether the death is peaceful. I remember a man in his late sixties who was dying from ALS. When he lost the ability to speak due to the disease, he wasn't able to communicate what he needed. Once he received a continuous-care nurse to help control his discomfort, he experienced some relief, but it was still a difficult death. Some diseases are just like that.

- **Personality or temperament:** If a person was very anxious and neurotic or angry and bitter in life, they'll likely leave the world the same way. Similarly, if someone was pretty chill or had a sunny disposition, they'll likely leave the world in the same way. People die how they lived.

Changes Just after Death

When a person has just died, their body will be noticeably different from how it was when they were living and healthy. Here are a few things you might notice:

- **Twitching:** You may see some twitching movements in the body after the person has died, which is normal. The chemical processes happening in the body can cause muscle contractions.

- **Skin color:** As when the person was actively dying, you likely will see some discoloration in the person's skin after death.

- **Slack jaw:** The jaw of the person who has died is often open, and their eyes may be as well.

- **Temperature:** After death, in most climates, the person's body will begin to cool, as the body's natural 98.6°F temperature drops to match the temperature in the room.

- **Stiffness:** At the end of life, a person's body may feel stiff or hard. If you try to move the limbs of the person who has died, they will feel particularly heavy.

- **Fluids and odor:** When the body dies, finally letting go, all the sphincters relax. This means that some people will release bowel movements or urine. You also may notice fluid being released from the sinuses or mouth.

All of these bodily responses are natural and normal. You're not required to clean up your loved one before the mortuary representative arrives. Only do what you're comfortable doing.

The Death Certificate

After your loved one dies, request multiple copies of the death certificate. You may not know yet all the various entities and agencies that may require a copy. As you sort out issues around property and finances, you'll need this document.

Death Is Not an Emergency

As caregivers, we learn to respond to the needs of our loved ones. When they let us know that they're hungry or thirsty, we get them food or drink. When they need pain relief, we offer it.

When our loved one dies, it's natural to feel the same impulse to *respond*. We might even feel a sense of urgency to do all the things we think we should do immediately: make the person look presentable, call the mortuary, call the hospice agency, care for the family and friends in our home, call other loved ones, and more. We might even feel a bit panicky.

Whether you're with your loved one when they die or you discover that they have died after the fact, there is nothing you have to do immediately. Simply notice that what has happened is sacred. Death is a natural part of life, and you have, in whatever way, participated in your loved one's journey toward this sacred moment. I want to give you the freedom, when your loved one dies, to pause and take a deep breath. Death is not an emergency. Nothing about this needs to be chaotic. There's no rush. There's nothing *urgent* you need to do when your loved one dies.

I encourage you to pause and pay attention to what's happening in you and around you. Notice the sense of stillness. Pause and be present in the moment. Notice what you feel and what you need. Take in the silence, or turn on music if you prefer.

At some point, you'll make the call for the body to be removed from the home.

Eventually, you'll phone everyone who needs to know.

Ultimately, you'll handle other responsibilities.

One day, you'll wash the sheets and make the bed.

But when the person you love dies, there's nothing that needs to be done immediately. Death is not an emergency. Give yourself the gift of pausing to be present.

Chapter 6

Deathbed Phenomena

When Juanita was evaluated to receive hospice care, she *barely* qualified. She was just on the borderline of being an appropriate candidate. She did have a terminal diagnosis—chronic obstructive pulmonary disorder (COPD)—that, if left untreated, would give her about six months to live, but she also seemed healthy and strong, considering. Importantly, however, she wasn't interested in receiving any treatments to extend her life. Our team signed off on her admission, but we knew it was possible she might continue doing well and ultimately have to come off hospice again. I was assigned to be her nurse.

Juanita was in her mid-eighties. She lived with her adult son, Ricky, who was fifty and had an intellectual disability. Their caretaker, Marianna, also lived in the home and had taken care of them both for several decades. When I visited them for Juanita's initial assessment, the love between the three of them was palpable. It also was clear to me that Juanita was not dying anytime soon. I completed my work but quietly wondered if she should be on hospice care at all.

So when I received a call the following week to let me know Juanita had died, I was shocked. I mean, I really couldn't believe it. I had *just* seen her, and she'd been doing really well. There had been no signs that she was near death.

When I got to the house midmorning, Marianna detailed the previous day for me. As they did every Sunday morning, Juanita and Marianna had made blueberry muffins together. After an afternoon nap, Juanita joined Ricky and Marianna for dinner. After they watched *Jeopardy!* on television, Marianna assisted her in getting cleaned up and ready for bed.

As Marianna helped her get settled, Juanita became sentimental and asked her to come close to her.

"Thank you so much for caring for me. I love you so much."

"I love you, too," Marianna said.

Juanita continued, "I'm really tired. I'm going to leave and go home."

"What are you talking about?" Marianna asked.

"I'm tired, and I'm going home," Juanita repeated.

Marianna reassured her, "Everything's fine, Juanita. You are home. I'll see you tomorrow."

"No, I'm really tired. I'm going home. Promise me that you'll take care of Ricky."

"Of course! I'll always take care of both of you. Stop talking like this."

Juanita asked Marianna to invite Ricky in to say goodnight.

When Ricky bent over to give his mother a goodnight kiss on the cheek, she reached up to squeeze his neck.

"I love you, sweet boy," she said. "And I'll always love you."

"I love you, too, Mom," he answered.

Shuffling Ricky out of the room, Marianna flipped off the light switch and carefully closed the door behind her.

The following morning, when Marianna opened the door to check on Juanita before breakfast, she discovered that Juanita had died peacefully in her sleep. It was as if she chose when she would die.

This is just one example of the fascinating, unexplainable things I've seen happen to dying people in hospice care. They're not rare occurrences either. Whether we're talking about visions, preknowledge of death, seeing bright lights or angels, or other phenomena, a significant number of dying people seem to experience such occurrences.

Medical professionals still can't adequately explain why most of these phenomena happen, but they occur so often that we actually put them in our hospice textbooks. Because whatever the cause, they *do* happen, they *are* a part of the dying process, and knowing about them helps us prepare both patients and their families. In medical and scientific texts, they are referred to as either death-related sensory experiences (DRSE) or simply deathbed phenomena (DBP).

Visioning

Visioning, also known as deathbed visions, is when a person who is dying begins to see people or things that aren't physically present in the room. If a dying person experiences visioning, it usually begins somewhere around three or four weeks before their death. These visions commonly can include the following:

- Deceased family members, such as parents, spouses, or siblings

- Other loved ones who have died, like grandparents, aunts, uncles, or friends

- Religious figures, such as angels, Jesus, Muhammad, or God

- Beloved pets who have died

- Beautiful landscapes or images

In addition to seeing these things, the dying person often will interact with them. They may hear a message, such as "We're coming to get you" or "Don't worry, we'll help." They might have a conversation with someone they're seeing. They might even reach out to touch whatever or whoever they believe to be in the room with them.

Sometimes they may ask others in the room if they're seeing the same vision and then describe what they're experiencing as it's happening. Or afterward, they'll talk about whom they encountered and what was said. At other times, the others in the room will have the privilege of listening to the dying person speak to a parent or loved one, although only the dying person can see them. Some patients might start talking about getting ready to go on a journey of some kind.

Typically, the kind of visioning a dying person experiences is related to who they are and their life experiences. If someone didn't like animals, they likely won't see a long-lost pet. Someone who had a horrible spouse often isn't going to see that person as the one warmly welcoming them to the other side. Someone who sees religious figures is likely a person of faith.

One man who lost his father shared that his dad hadn't been close with his parents, so they weren't the ones to welcome him to the afterlife. But in his final days, the father did encounter a beloved family dog who'd died years earlier. He told his adult children that the dog was curled up at the end of his bed. With a smile on his face, the son told me that totally made sense for who his dad was.

So although it's possible that someone could have a visioning experience that's completely foreign to who they are, that's not how it usually goes. We typically see an agreement between who the person was while living and who they are while dying. Our inner character doesn't change suddenly at the end of life.

I see visioning as much as 80 percent of the time in the dying. It happens so often that our agency addresses it in the educational package we give to the families of our patients so that they can understand it when they see it. It's important for loved ones to know that visioning is common and harmless, and that the person having the experience usually isn't afraid at all—in fact, in nearly all cases, medical professionals report that these visions have a calming effect, helping the patient feel more peaceful in their final days before death.

What I also find interesting is that, most of the time, my hospice patients who have these experiences *know* that the person they're seeing is dead. They're not in an altered state where they think the person is alive and in the room, and they're often just as curious as I am! They're alert and oriented when it's happening, fully understanding that no one else can see or hear what they're seeing and hearing. (Of course, if someone is already in an altered mental state, then they may not be able to communicate to us whether or not they know the person is dead.)

I once had a patient named Julio, an older gentleman. On the day I went to visit him, he was completely lucid. He was not yet in the process of actively dying, and he was very clear mentally.

When Julio's daughters stepped out of the room, he grabbed my arm to make sure he had my attention. "I've been seeing my parents," he said. "My parents came to me and told me that I was going to go with them soon and not to worry."

He sounded as if he was ashamed of what he'd witnessed.

"What was that like for you?" I asked him.

He said, still a bit sheepishly, "Well, before, I was afraid of dying. But now I'm not." He seemed to want some reassurance.

"This is very, very normal," I said. "As long as you feel good about it, don't worry. It's totally okay. I see this all the time." I left the room and joined his family in the kitchen.

His daughter Emilia looked very concerned. "He needs medication. He's been saying he's seeing his parents, but his parents are dead. He's really confused."

Now I understood why he'd waited until they left the room

to share this with me. His family hadn't believed him, or at best, had misunderstood him.

I used the opportunity to gently educate them. I let them know that what their father and grandfather was experiencing wasn't confusion at all, but rather a fairly typical experience for those who are dying—in fact, probably the most commonly reported and discussed deathbed phenomenon. These types of visions have been reported across all countries and cultures and throughout recorded history. This is not at all a new occurrence.

As an ICU nurse, I often witnessed people with delirium, psychosis, and hallucinations, and I can tell you that they behaved very differently from the people I've seen having deathbed visions. Delirium, psychosis, and hallucinations usually come with serious agitation and restlessness, while deathbed visions come with peace and well-being. From what I've seen, these visions always seem to be soothing and reassuring, giving the patient a sense of comfort, love, and care in their final days.

The Death Stare

Closely related to visioning is another phenomenon that is more physically visible to those in the room with the dying person. It's called the "death stare" or the "death reach." About one or two weeks before death, a dying person will sometimes begin to look past everyone, staring at the wall, the ceiling, the corner of the room, or somewhere far off in the distance. They often won't look away from that point for a long time. This staring is often accompanied by the person lifting their arms, reaching out to something or someone.

Sometimes both of these things happen together, and some-

Ginny's Last Request

As a hospice nurse, I get the privilege of hearing some of the most amazing stories from the people I serve. This one gave me chills.

Helen shared with me that she had been taking care of her mother, Ginny, in the months leading up to her death. Despite being fairly unresponsive, when Ginny would wake up from sleep, she'd yell the names of her siblings and tell them to come open the door for her. "Curtis, I'm outside. Come open this door!" "Dorothy, let me in!" "Roland, open the door!"

When this behavior began, Helen would open the door to the bedroom to see if that was what her mother wanted. Then she'd open the door to the closet and to the bathroom. But nothing helped. Meanwhile, Ginny, who seemed sort of agitated, would continue to request, "Would you open a door for me?"

"Where were her siblings?" I asked, wondering if they lived nearby or far away.

"That's the thing," Helen said. "All of her siblings were dead. She was the last one alive out of ten children."

That's when I began to catch on.

Helen shared that when her mother finally died, she had the thought, "I think they came to open that door."

I think so, too.

times they happen separately. On several occasions, I've witnessed dying patients staring off at a distant point and smiling broadly, or reaching out at nothing and smiling.

When they're reaching or staring, many of these patients also might say something like, "Don't you see it?" or "It's so beautiful!" When the person is able to speak and tell us what's going on, we might label their experience as visioning. When they're not able to speak and we don't know if a vision accompanies the behavior or not, we call it the death stare or death reach. In both cases, the dying person is connecting to a world beyond this one in a way that the rest of us can't perceive.

Reports from the Other Side

You've probably read about people who have had incredible near-death experiences. Maybe they briefly died on an operating table and felt themselves drift up and out of their bodies, able to see from above everything that was happening in the operating room. Or perhaps they stopped breathing for a significant amount of time, and when they were finally revived, they described an encounter with a beautiful world that they could only describe as "heaven." What happens at and after death are well-guarded secrets, yet these rare, remarkable reports let us imagine what might be coming after we die.

But people don't necessarily need to be miraculously revived to experience the unusual. Those of us who accompany someone during their journey through the process of dying often are privileged to get these eyewitness reports of someplace "else."

These otherworldly experiences occur just as often in those dying at home, in bed, surrounded by family and caregivers. There doesn't seem to be a special pass required to experience a nearness to the other side.

When one woman asked her dying mother, who seemed to be fixated on staring at one spot in the room, what she was seeing, her mother smiled and whispered, "Light."

One man shared that his dying father reported, "The table is set, and it's beautiful."

Minutes before one woman's mother died, she reached up for her husband, who'd died five years earlier. "Oh, Bob," she said, "I've missed you so much." When she lowered her arms, she began to cry. Then she said, "Bob, I'm coming," before she slipped away, holding the hand of her daughter.

One woman said that her dad had a huge picture of Jesus on the wall in the living room. One day he instructed, "Take that picture down. He looks nothing like that." He died three days later.

Another person reported that her mother had been unresponsive for days, but right before she died, she said, "Oh, the light. It's just so beautiful."

The father of one man had died back in the 1960s. At his wife's request, he'd been fixing a household appliance, and she'd been serving as his helper. He asked her to plug in the appliance, and when she did, he was electrocuted and died. For years, this woman carried the guilt of believing she'd been responsible for her husband's death. Her son was her caregiver in her later years, and when she was on her deathbed, he reported that although she was mostly unresponsive, right before she died, she seemed to have a burst of cognition. In his words, "She lit up like a Christmas tree." Looking directly at the ceiling, her face exuded joy as if she was seeing someone she hadn't seen in years. Her son is confident that she saw her husband coming to get her and greeting her with open arms.

Do I understand everything that's happening with these reports? Not at all. Do I know why they happen? I don't. What I do know is that whatever they are, they happen and they're important—not because they might offer some proof of life after death, or angels, or spirits, but because they show over and over again that *death can be peaceful.* They show that our loved ones aren't suffering as they die. On the contrary, many of them are having beautiful visions, meeting with long-dead loved ones, or having spiritual experiences in line with their deeply held beliefs.

I don't know if these experiences prove there's an afterlife, but I do think they prove that death can be beautiful and is not something to be feared.

I don't know if these experiences prove there's an afterlife, but I do think they prove that death can be beautiful and is not something to be feared.

The Rally

Although I wasn't present when my grandmother died, my mom described for me what happened. It was Thanksgiving, and my grandmother, who was close to death, hadn't been eating. But my mom still brought her a plate of Thanksgiving dinner, just in case. When my mom walked into my grandmother's room, my grandma was standing next to the bed and said to my mom, "Let's go!"

My mom was absolutely shocked because my grandmother hadn't spoken or stood up in days—let alone walked around. Besides, there was a snowstorm outside, so they weren't going anywhere. My mom said to her, "There's a storm out there, so why don't we sit down here and eat Thanksgiving dinner?" (She had to yell because my grandmother couldn't hear well at the end.)

To my mother's great surprise, Grandma wanted to eat. She even gave my mom attitude about the food not being hot enough as she ate. It made my mom so happy to see her grumpy, sassy mother back the way she used to be. They ate Thanksgiving dinner together and then grandma got back into bed and didn't get up again. She died a few days later.

This phenomenon, known as the "rally," happens in about 30 percent of dying patients. It also can be referred to as the "surge," and the technical language for it is "terminal lucidity." I like to think of it as a patient's last hurrah. When it happens, we see a person who's been declining experience a burst of uncharacteristic energy. The rally can last anywhere from a few minutes to a few hours to a few days. They may look better, get up and walk around, talk to their family or caregiver, or eat a meal.

During the rally, the dying patient may get their old personality back, become their sarcastic self again, make a joke, or tell stories. Family members might say, "He seems like his old self again." This period is marked by mental alertness that may not have been present in the weeks or even months beforehand. Even in patients who have been affected by degenerative diseases, a return of cognitive functions can happen for a short time.

The rally is different from someone who's ill and just happens to have a good day. After the rally, the patient returns to their former condition and dies soon afterward. If this sort of resurgence lasts longer than a few days, it's not a rally, and something else is going on.

This is why education about the topic of death is so important. If families aren't educated about what might occur, this surge of energy or mental clarity in their loved one can give families false hope that they might recover. When the person then dies soon after, it can be a shock, even though it shouldn't be. The family just didn't know how to interpret the signs.

Health care professionals don't definitively know why the rally happens in so many patients. I find the rally to be a massive gift. The families get to experience their loved ones one last time, and patients get to put any final things in order or say any last words before death arrives. When we can recognize the rally for what it is, we're able to enjoy it for as long as it lasts. It doesn't happen for everyone, but for many people, the rally is a normal part of death and dying.

Choosing When to Die

There are some people, like Juanita from earlier in this chapter, who just know when they're going to die. I don't know how they know, but they know. There are others, far less lucid than Juanita, who even seem to *choose* when they'll die. Of course, not everyone appears to have control over their time of death, but when they do, I often see one of three things happen:

1. The person waits to die until every last one of their family members or friends arrives to be present with them.

2. The person waits to die until every last family member or friend leaves the room or the house.

3. The person waits to die until after a milestone has occurred.

All of these scenarios are so common in my experience, and I've seen each of them play out many, many times. Let's take a closer look at them.

The Person Dies When Everyone Has Arrived

Sometimes a person will wait until all of their loved ones have flown or driven in from other places to say goodbye before they die. Or they'll wait for every person to be physically present in the room with them and then they'll let go. This most often happens with a person who's social and extroverted, who thrives off the energy of others.

Rachel had turned one hundred just five months before I met her when she came on hospice. At that time, a huge crowd of children, grandchildren, great-grandchildren, and even a few great-great-grandchildren gathered to celebrate the life of the family matriarch.

When I evaluated Rachel, it was very evident that she was in the stage of actively dying. All the signs were there. I saw it in the pallor of her skin. I heard it in her breathing. I noticed it in her lack of interest in or ability to eat food. The end was near.

"So," I explained to Rachel's two daughters who were in the home when I stopped by to do the admission. "What I'm seeing is that she's actively dying. That means that in the next few days, she'll die. So whoever needs to be here, get them here."

Nodding, the sisters, who were in their seventies, agreed to mobilize everyone who'd want to come and say goodbye to Rachel.

Over the following two or three days, family members flooded into Rachel's home to say goodbye. Although she was unresponsive, I was still glad to see the love that was surrounding her. When one of Rachel's daughters told me that one of the grandchildren couldn't make it from New Jersey until the following week, I knew she'd get there too late to say goodbye to Rachel. But maybe she'd be there in time for the funeral service.

When I came to the house a week after I'd predicted Rachel had just two or three days to live, I met this granddaughter. I was very surprised Rachel had lasted a week. A week later, another grandchild, living in a different part of the state, who hadn't even planned on coming, had a three-day weekend and showed up to say his final goodbyes. How Rachel had lasted two weeks, fully unconscious, without food or water, baffled me. Whenever I'd visit, I could hear Rachel's daughters giving her updates about who still wanted to come to say goodbye to her, and Rachel *kept living*.

In the end, Rachel lasted seventeen days in that state of actively dying, without food or water. Just hours after the final family member came to say goodbye, Rachel finally let go. I'd never seen anything like it. Rachel absolutely decided when she was going to die.

The Person Dies When Everyone Has Left

Conversely, some people wait until their loved ones have left their bedside before dying. Sometimes these family members have kept vigil for hours or days, yet it's when they finally step away that the person dies. Whether they leave to go home and rest for the night or just step out to grab a cup of coffee, *that's* when the person—often someone who's more private or introverted, who prefers time alone—dies.

When someone chooses to die when no one's around, family members have confessed to me that they feel guilty, as if somehow they've failed their loved one by not being present with them in the actual moment of their death. They might wonder, "Is he punishing us?" or "Is she trying to get back at me for something?" No. Likely not. This is just something they needed to do for their own dying process. Much like in life, in death, a person's behavior isn't usually about us, but about them and what they need. If we imagine that the person who is dying was "holding on" in some way for the sake of those in the room, then giving the person the space and solitude they need to let go is the most gracious thing we can do for them. I don't think anyone who's spent any kind of time with the person who's dying should feel guilty for not being present at their last breath. It's likely that that is exactly how the dying person wanted it to be. When this happens, you can take comfort knowing that it's what *they* needed.

Take Walter. Walter's wife made four phone calls to alert the couple's four children that their father, who'd been on hospice care for months, likely would die within one or two days. In a scramble to book last-minute plane tickets, all four adults were able to make their way home to be with their father in his final days.

Walter was showing many of the signs that let me know death was near. For days, he'd been eating and drinking less. He had become unconscious and unresponsive. His breathing had become irregular, and I detected the raspy death rattle. His pale skin had become mottled in places, and his body temperature was fluctuating. Walter was a textbook case of someone who is actively dying.

The day after Walter's wife had alerted her children to his impending death, they'd all dragged in chairs from the dining room to be seated around him as he died. Among the five of them, they worked out a schedule so that Walter would never be alone—so that he wouldn't die alone. One day of this vigil became two. Two became three. On the fourth day, a longtime neighbor brought over a small feast, around lunchtime, to feed the family. Although Walter's wife had been stationed at his bedside, when she heard the doorbell, she scrambled to the kitchen to put plates, cups, and utensils on the table.

When the family was halfway through the meal, one of them remarked, "Dad would *love* this mac and cheese."

And that's when they realized that Walter was alone.

When one of his children hopped up to check on him, she returned quickly to let her family know that Walter had died. Sometimes people wait to be alone to let go.

The Person Dies after a Milestone

Sometimes a person chooses a date with personal significance—a holiday, wedding, birthday, or anniversary—and dies on that day. "I'm going to wait until after my grandson is born." "I'm going to make it to my eighty-eighth birthday." Then, they let go. Although not everyone is able to achieve it, I've seen many people who will hang on with a vengeance to make it to a special milestone. I've noticed that these people are often the ones who are very willful or independent (aka stubborn), as well as those who have deep connections to tradition or specific anniversaries that shaped their lives.

Mitzy, one of my followers on social media, shared this amazing story with me: Her mother was on hospice while Mitzy's daughter was nine months pregnant. Mitzy was sitting in a chair beside her mom's bed, reading, when she received a phone call that her daughter, who lived in another state, was having contractions. Mitzy was torn.

"Mom, I don't know what to do," Mitzy told her mother, who was still lucid. "I don't want to leave you. I'm afraid if I leave, something's going to happen, but I do want to see my grandson being born."

With confidence, Mitzy's mother assured her, "Honey, you have to go. If you don't, you're going to regret it. Don't worry about me. I'm going to stay here until your grandson is born."

Although Mitzy was conflicted about her decision, she took her mother's advice and drove several hours to be with her daughter. When Mitzy checked in with her brother from the road a few hours into her trip, he reported that as soon as Mitzy left, their mother seemed to go into a deep sleep.

Late that night, after Mitzy arrived at her daughter's home, they discovered that her contractions had not, in fact, meant that she was in labor. Instead, they were "false alarm" contractions called Braxton-Hicks. No labor. No grandson.

The following morning, Mitzy drove straight back home to be at her mother's side. Even though her mother was unresponsive, Mitzy narrated the trip for her, explaining that the baby had not yet come. Then she remembered her mother's promise.

Gently, with kind assurance, Mitzy whispered in her mother's ear, "It's okay, Mom. You can go. It's okay."

But her mother held on.

A whole week later, her mother was still unresponsive. When Mitzy's daughter went into legitimate active labor, Mitzy repeated her trip to be with her daughter and welcome her grandson.

After the baby's birth, Mitzy phoned her mother's home and asked her brother to put the phone to her mother's ear.

"Mom, we have a healthy grandson. He has ten fingers and ten toes! Everything went great."

Mitzy's brother called her back fifteen minutes later to let her know that their mother had died. The family would always joke that Mitzy's mother and the grandbaby high-fived each other, one entering this world as the other was exiting.

The Behavior of Pets

It's not just people who experience seemingly supernatural phenomena. Sometimes our *pets* seem to connect to another world as well.

The daughter of a hospice patient told me that as her father was dying, he and his dog *both* kind of fixated on a particular corner of the room for a week before he died. Just stared at that corner, together. It was as if the dog could see exactly what his owner was seeing, whatever that might have been.

At other times, a pet will seem to take on the same symptoms the owner is experiencing. One woman who was accompanying her husband through his dying process told me that she had to keep taking their dog to the vet. He was acting lethargic, no longer wanted to go out on walks, and even was vomiting. But visit after visit, the vet couldn't find anything wrong with the dog. In conversation, they finally realized that the dog was mimicking the symptoms of his owner. The dog was being super protective and would never leave the owner's side. If he wasn't snuggled up against the owner *on* the bed, he was tucked right under it.

And although those kinds of extreme occurrences in animals aren't common, what we see often is that a pet will behave in a very protective way around their dying owner. They refuse to leave their owner's side. They may lie on the bed with the person who is dying, or they might lie under it. Just like people can experience something beyond this world, it appears that our pets also can be in touch with the beyond.

Why I Don't Fear Death

When we talk about deathbed phenomena, we're usually referring to the experiences of the dying person, but caregivers often have inexplicable, seemingly miraculous experiences, too. One of the big reasons I don't fear death is because of such experiences I've had with my patients. Now, believe me, I'm not saying that I'm looking forward to death or that I have any definite ideas about what comes after. But as far as the process of dying is concerned, I feel really confident that it's going to be okay. I'm not scared of suffering or being in pain or having anxiety. As I've seen others dying, I've seen them experience such peace.

One of these patients was Randy. Randy was and still is one of my favorite patients. He was dying of pancreatic cancer at a young age, and when he came to hospice, he was struggling. He was also a hoarder. Hoarding is a disorder in which people have difficulty parting with possessions, to the point that their surroundings can become very cramped and even dangerous. When Randy became our patient, he was living in unsafe conditions, an apartment literally *filled* from top to bottom with stuff. On top of that, Randy had severe social anxiety. He didn't have support, and I knew he would need a lot of it. Our amazing social worker was immediately there to help. We had a meeting and decided we had to help him either drastically clean his place or move. Randy had been alone for so long and had needed help for so long, I think that by the time we got there, he was ready. Thankfully.

He didn't hesitate. He said yes to the help and allowed us to call his distant cousins to come for the weekend. About a week later, when I visited, I couldn't believe my eyes. It was like he had a new apartment. He had been able to let go of so much. He looked like a brand-new person, too, like a weight had been lifted off him. He was so happy to have his "mess" cleaned up. He told me he thought it was ironic that it took a terminal illness to make him feel alive again.

Randy ended up living much longer than we had expected, around eight or nine months. During that time, we spent many visits just talking. We talked about his childhood, his time in the military, and his family. We both liked the big, deep questions: "What do you think happens after we die?" "Should I be afraid?" "Where do you think we go?" Randy thought a lot, and although he was finding comfort in his new friends from the hospice team, he still had a lot of fear about dying. Our team helped him physically, emotionally, and spiritually. We all felt truly connected to Randy; he was our patient but also had become our friend.

During his active dying phase, Randy developed terminal agitation. This is fairly normal at the end of life, and we were able to get him a continuous-care nurse to be with him twenty-four hours a day. I would visit him every day during that time, and on one of my visits, I could tell he was very close to death.

I stood over his bed, closed my eyes, and quietly said, "Randy, I love you, and thank you for all you've given me. I'll miss you and hope you find all your answers."

I left after that, telling his continuous-care nurse to text or call me when he died. I went to my car and sat there for a minute, just taking a moment. I was sad but also happy for him. I said one last prayer: "God, help our sweet friend die peacefully."

Moments later, I heard Randy's voice clear as day in my head. I suddenly felt this intense feeling of relief and freedom. It was the most exuberant feeling you could ever imagine. Just intense joy. I couldn't help but weep. As I sat in my car, I continued to hear Randy's voice. He was saying, "Oh my gosh, Julie. Oh my gosh, Julie. I can't believe this. I can't believe how good it is. If I had only known. I couldn't have known how good it is. I can't believe it."

As I was hearing this, I could *feel* what he was feeling—the freedom, the peace, the joy. I was so overwhelmed by the feeling of *home*. It was the most unbelievable, unimaginable experience. All of this happened within thirty seconds and then stopped as quickly as it started. I heard my phone beep. The nurse inside Randy's house had texted me: *Randy died.*

I thought to myself, "I know. I think he just showed me."

I didn't tell anyone what had happened for a while because I was scared of sounding weird. But this experience is one of the reasons why I really don't have a fear of dying. Randy's visit was so real in that moment. It was so pure and so amazing. Whatever's going to happen to me when I die, I know it's going to be good. Because if anyone wasn't sure about that, it was this guy, and he showed me that he was okay.

The Pancakes Story

Randy's is the only "shared death" experience I've had, but I've had other experiences that felt just as miraculous.

One night we got a late hospice admission, and I'll be honest: I felt irritated at first because I didn't want to work late. (This was early in my career, before I learned how to set better personal boundaries in my nursing work, but that's another story!) Regardless, when I got the call, I responded quickly, "Yes, I'll be right there."

I arrived at the house just as an ambulance pulled up to drop off the patient from the hospital. I walked up, went inside, and saw the patient lying on the stretcher, and to my eyes, she was actively dying. After an initial check, I believed she was only hours or days away from dying. As the EMTs got the woman settled in her bed, I looked around the room at her children. They were all young adults in their early twenties, obviously concerned about their mother and anxious for what was likely right around the corner.

They immediately started asking me questions like, "When can we start physical therapy?" and "How long until she'll be walking again?" As I stood there, doing my best to field these questions honestly but at the same time compassionately, my heart sank. They had no idea what was really happening. No one at the hospital had told them their mom was dying, or if they had been told, they hadn't heard it.

So I sat them down next to their mother, who by this point was lying peacefully on the bed and still showing clear signs of actively dying.

"What do you know about your mother's disease?" I asked them.

They stared blankly at me.

Then one of the kids spoke up. "We know it's bad, but she's gotten worse in the hospital. She'll be better now that she's home. We just need to get her walking again, and eating again, to get her strength up."

It's common for families not to fully understand or appreciate what is happening with their loved one. Normally, when I sense this is happening, I like to explain how I know what I know. So I started to share how long I'd been a nurse, how many times I'd seen a patient like their mother, and what I knew specifically about her disease. Then I gave them a brief description of where their mother was in the progression of the disease. I began pointing out the symptoms I had noticed.

"I've been doing this a long time, and I have to tell you, I think your mother is getting close to the end of her life," I said finally.

I also pointed out to them that their mother appeared very comfortable, which is always ideal but was another sign that death was likely very near. I showed them her changes in breathing, her unresponsiveness, and her changes in skin color, all signs of impending death.

They seemed to understand. I said that if there were any additional family members or friends that they wanted to call, now was the time. They began calling family members, and I started to change the mother's hospital gown and sheets, making sure she was comfortable and clean. Afterward, I called the family into her room so they could spend time with her. I told them that her death was coming soon.

I spent a long time at the house that night, organizing everything and making sure the children would have what they needed for their mother medically. I believed her death was so imminent that I would still be there when she died. She had mottling on her fingers and toes, her lips were purple and blue, and she experienced significant breathing changes. After more than an hour of being there, I decided to go home. I didn't want to leave, only for the on-call nurse to have to come right out for a death visit a few minutes later. (Nurses are always thinking of each other.) But it was getting late, the patient was comfortable, and her kids were okay, so I left. Before I did, I told them, "Please call us if anything happens, and when she dies, please call us, and we'll come right out."

At home that night, I couldn't stop thinking of the family, hoping the mother would have a peaceful death and that her kids would be okay. I finally went to bed, knowing that she would be dead by the morning.

The next day, I woke and checked my email first thing. There were no emails about her death or another nurse's death visit overnight. I thought that was weird, but I guessed they simply hadn't sent the email yet. As the morning went on, still nothing came through, and my curiosity got the better of me.

I called the office and asked, "Hey, who attended the death visit for our late admit last night?"

The office worker sounded confused. "There were no death calls last night . . . did someone die?"

Now I was confused. No death calls? I hung up the phone and immediately called the family, afraid that maybe they had panicked and called 911 instead of us. The son answered the phone, and he sounded happy.

"Oh, hi, Julie!" he said.

"Hi. How are you guys doing? Everything okay?"

"Yes, everything is great over here. Mom's just up having pancakes."

My jaw dropped. Awake? Up? Alive? Eating? *Pancakes?* Now, of course, I didn't say any of these things into the phone. I just said, "Wow! Wonderful! Do you mind if I stop by?" I needed to see this with my own eyes!

When I got to the house, there she was, sitting at the table, eating pancakes, smiling, talking, walking around. Never in my fifteen years of nursing had I seen someone make such a massive comeback after being so incredibly close to death.

My mind tried to understand and explain this scientifically. There is, as I've discussed, a phenomenon called the "rally" or the "surge" in which someone who is close to death looks well for a day or two and gains more energy but then dies shortly after. I figured that must be what was happening here. As much as I didn't want to be the bearer of bad news, I did make sure to educate the family about this phenomenon that was likely happening to their mother.

But it turned out I was wrong again. Their mother lived another three months, fully walking, talking, eating, and enjoying her children until the end.

I truly believe that I witnessed a minor miracle, seeing her life go on that long after observing how close she was to dying earlier. There's no explanation for this occurrence and no reasonable rationale that I can point to. But I did eventually tell the family that I believed their mother was a miracle, and they felt the same about getting all that additional time with their mother at the end of her life.

I love sharing this story, but there's another part to it that I didn't tell for a long time. That first night that I visited, her kids were in the other room calling family members to let them know their mom was dying. When I went in to check on this woman who was actively dying, I got this sudden vision of what I guess I would consider to be an angel.

I don't know what angels are or what they look like, but this wasn't what you would think an angel would look like. In my mind's eye, it was this huge being—not at all like the cute baby cherubs on greeting cards. It was this huge, massive thing that seemed to be standing over this woman's bed. I quickly pushed it out of my mind and didn't think about it again that night because I don't know anything about that stuff.

The next day, when I visited the family, you'll recall that I was surprised she hadn't died the previous night. That's when my mind went back to the vision I had of this being standing over her bed. It wasn't a scary thing. It was a large, beautiful, angelic thing.

It's hard for me to know how to talk about this sort of thing because I don't live in the realm of fully believing in angels, or of fully understanding what I witnessed. I even doubt myself sometimes because I'm such a skeptic. But I'll try to describe it to you.

I didn't see it with my eyes, like I'm seeing my computer screen right now as I write this. It was like a vision in my mind's eye and then a feeling. One thing I saw was this very large solid block full of shapes, all the way to the ceiling, if not higher. It was as wide as a car and solid. It felt like solid brick. And it did give me the sense that it had wings, but they were tucked back, so you couldn't see them but knew they were there.

If you're Catholic, you may remember that old-school Mother Mary statue, where she's standing in a long blue dress and a blue veil. It was almost like that—but definitely not Mother Mary. It did not give me that vibe. But it was kind of a solid block in the same way. It was cream-colored and leaning over the patient's bed. There were no facial features. It felt just *dominant*— powerful, secure, strong.

It wasn't scary at all, but it also didn't feel loving or soft. It felt like *power*. If it could speak, it would say, "I got this."

I had the sense that this thing didn't care about me being there. It was more like, "My main focus is to be with this person in bed. She's mine."

Did I see an angel? I don't know. It all happened within seconds. The next morning, I was asking myself, "Did I really see that?" But when I saw this woman the next morning, eating *pancakes*, I had to wonder. I think I did.

What Science Says

When I share these kinds of stories, I still feel slightly embarrassed. Even though I've got a few stories, these mystical experiences are very atypical for me. Let me be clear that I'm all about the science and physiology of dying. I have a medical understanding of each of the signs we see when someone is actively dying. Biologically, each of those *makes sense*. I understand why they're happening, and I'm grateful that they happen.

But these end-of-life phenomena are a different story. Seeing dead people? Reaching for something that's not there? Being near death and then eating pancakes? Deciding when to die? I'm not even going to pretend that I understand how and why these things happen to those who are near death.

Science, too, doesn't really understand what's happening in people's bodies when these seemingly mystical things occur. But we may be getting closer to answers.

While a team of scientists were studying the brainwaves of a patient who'd developed epilepsy, he suddenly suffered a fatal heart attack. Although they weren't expecting it, the scientists were able to learn something from this unique experience. When they looked at the brainwave patterns in the thirty seconds before and after the patient's death, they saw that they followed the same patterns as someone who was dreaming or recalling memories. One of the coauthors of the study they published told the BBC, "This could possibly be a last recall of memories that we've experienced in life, and they replay through our brain in the last seconds before we die."

If this is true, it resonates with phenomena like visioning, the death stare, and the death reach. This idea of memories we have from life somehow connecting to another world really aligns with the kinds of experiences patients on hospice have as they're dying.

This is scientifically interesting, of course, but in the end, I think it is unimportant. If your loved one is having experiences like these, I encourage you to notice how they are *affected* by the experience. That's the important thing to me. Do these experiences—real or not, science or science-fiction—comfort, soothe, calm, or reassure the dying person? If you're hesitant to believe that something real and meaningful is happening in your loved one who is dying, notice what the effect is on them. If it's positive, then just go with it. Notice how it helps.

The stories I've told in this chapter are simply things I've experienced. I love them partly because, whatever their origin, they make the experience of death so much richer. Mostly I like them because they bring up questions, and questions are good. When we ask questions about death, we become familiar with it and get less afraid.

As much as we'd like to, we simply don't understand everything about these encounters. They're mysteries. For my part, I can say that my own few experiences have given me nothing but confidence that a better world awaits us. I *do* believe that there's an afterlife because of experiences like these.

Having witnessed so many deaths, I feel like I've had the privilege of seeing a veil being lifted as people are on their way to a place that feels like home. Obviously, there's sadness, too, because people are grieving and losing a loved one. But watching the body take care of itself and feeling the energy in the room *change* after someone dies . . . if you can remain present, it can feel sacred.

In many ways, it feels a lot like the wonder of birth. When I get to see a baby being born, I weep from joy. I look at that baby and wonder, "Where did you come from?" When someone dies, I have that same feeling I get when babies are born. It's a feeling of *home*. Of comfort. I sense that it's a place I already know. When a baby is born, there's an undeniable feeling of "That was magical!" That is how it can feel when you see someone taking their last breath.

Since I was a little girl, I've always felt homesick for a place that I couldn't quite remember, and now I think I understand why. I think that when we die, we awaken in a place we've always known but had forgotten.

Chapter 7

Advice for the Dying

Not everybody gets the chance to know when they're going to die. But there are certain situations, such as with terminal diagnoses, when we do know, more or less. If you're in such a situation, the best thing you can do for yourself is to ask yourself how you want to die. Because if you know how you want to die, it will help you decide, with the time you have left, how you want to *live*.

Of course, there are some things you won't know. There are some things you can't control. But it's important that you understand one thing clearly: You get to decide how you live and how you die. You're the boss of this operation. If you know you're going to die from a terminal illness, you get to choose, to a degree, how you want that to unfold. I want to encourage you to pause and think about how you want *your* journey to unfold.

You get to decide how you live and how you die.

It's also important that you know it's not over until it's over. *You're not dead yet.* I'm serious. While you're living, you can choose to live your best life, however that might look. Will it be all that you want it to be? Maybe not. Will you suffer losses as your journey unfolds? Yes. But you also can choose how to walk this path.

It's awful to be dying of a disease you did not choose. That choice was out of your hands. But although there are profound losses at the end of life, I challenge you to embrace the gifts that a prepared death can give you.

When you know that you're dying—whether in six months, six weeks, or six days—you have the opportunity to be intentional about how you use your time. You get to choose what these last months, weeks, and days on your journey include. Here are a few ideas to get you started:

- Do the self-growth work you want to do to accept your death.

- Tell your family and friends that you love them.

- Ask forgiveness from people you've hurt.

- Exercise healthy boundaries around your space, which might mean excluding people who may be harmful to you.

- Ask yourself what brings you the most joy and then do it.

Whatever you do, be intentional. This is *your* end-of-life journey.

Accept Help

In our society, we're taught to be independent, rugged, and self-sufficient. I know I was. We think that we can and should do things by ourselves, that we don't—and shouldn't—need others. There are times when this attitude serves us well. The end of life is not one of those times.

Right now, *you need community*. You need help. If you've been trying not to be a "burden" to your family and friends, I'd like to help you think about it differently. This moment is *sacred*. It also may be lots of other things, like scary and painful and messy. But it's also sacred. This moment deserves respect and reverence.

The people who love you want to be a part of it. Yes, they may be limited by other responsibilities in their lives. Yes, it may be inconvenient at times. But I'm telling you, they want to be there for you. I know this because *they have told me*. In messages and in comments and in person, again and again, I am told by people that they want to be *more* involved in their loved one's death, not less. Please allow your family and other loved ones to be there for you. *Let your people love you.*

I once had a patient named Pearl. She was older and dying of terminal cancer. She had been doing very well for several weeks. One day I made my usual visit to see her. Her door was unlocked, which always makes me nervous because you never know what you're going to find entering an unlocked house alone. But I had been here before, and I knew that Pearl lived with her sister, who was her primary caretaker. Things were likely all right.

When I entered, however, things were not all right. Pearl was alone, sitting in a chair in the living room. Because Pearl had been doing so well, her sister had decided to go on vacation for a week. Unfortunately, this was the very week that Pearl's body chose to decline.

She couldn't get up or move around. Couldn't go to the bathroom, couldn't get her own food or water. I asked her if there was anybody else who could come and help her today. She told me that her grandson was coming over after work that night.

It was only eleven a.m.

I wouldn't be able to stay with her all day. I did what I could. I cleaned her and made her comfortable. I went and got her some lunch. As we were sitting talking and eating, her grandson called. The phone was near the chair, and she picked it up. I heard them chatting. It was obvious that they had a good relationship. Suddenly, I became aware that she was saying things like, "No, honey, I'm fine." "I can manage on my own until then." "I have everything I need." And then she hung up!

Pearl literally was unable to get out of her chair to go to the bathroom, and here she was telling her loving grandson who called to check up on her that she was just fine.

I made her call her grandson right back, and I spoke with him to explain the situation. Not only did he leave work immediately to come to her side, he also called other friends and family. Soon she was surrounded by loved ones. We even managed to get ahold of her sister on vacation. She wanted to come home, and we were able to get her a ticket through an organization called Give a Mile that arranges free flights for family members of the dying. (See the Resources in the back of the book for more information.)

Pearl was in tears, thanking me over and over again for the help that I'd gotten her. But I hadn't done a thing, other than encourage her to ask for help. Pearl had a huge network of people who loved and adored her. All Pearl had to do was ask, but she'd simply been too afraid.

Pearl had not been okay. Her decline was real, and she died that week, surrounded by family and loved ones, thanks to the fact that she finally allowed them to help.

Like so many other parts of this journey toward death, your need for people to care for you is going to happen whether you want it to or not. The two choices you have are to resist it or to allow it.

If you *resist* the care offered to you by family and friends, it may look and sound like this:

"I can do it myself."

"Don't worry about visiting. I know you're busy."

"I'm so sorry you have to do this."

"I hate being such a burden."

If you *allow* the care offered to you by family and friends, it may look and sound like this:

"I need and appreciate your help."

"If you're able to visit, I'd love to spend time with you."

"Thank you."

"I'm grateful for your care."

Step out of your body for a moment and imagine yourself on the "helper" end of the equation. Would you rather your loved one resisted your help, or would you rather they allowed it? Don't resist the care your family and friends want to give you—not just for your own sake, but for theirs.

Because, let me remind you, this is happening. Your death is happening, and receiving care from others is happening. You are the person who gets to set the tone for how it will happen. If a coworker offers to bring a meal, accept it. If a neighbor offers to spend time with you so that your primary caregivers can get out of the house, welcome them. If a friend is willing to give you a bath, let that friend help.

Practice receiving what is offered to you with gratitude.

Use Your Resources

If you're in hospice care, a number of people are at your disposal. (See chapter 3 for more details about each of these roles and how they can help you.) Please take advantage of them. Let these people know what you need. They include but may not be limited to the following:

- A hospice doctor

- A hospice nurse

- A hospice social worker

- A hospice chaplain

- A home health aide

- Volunteers

- A bereavement specialist

You also should have personal resources available to you. There is no reason for you to be alone. Use the resources that are at your disposal! These could include the following:

- **Your family:** If you have family with you, allow them to care for you. Although it may feel counterintuitive, it's a gift *you* give to *them*.

- **Your friends:** Let your friends love you, too. They want to care for you, and they might not know how best to do that. Do you want them to bring you takeout to share for dinner? Do you want them to come over and watch TV with you? Or read a favorite book together out loud? Let them know how you want them to take care of you.

- **Others:** Beyond your closest friends and family, there are others who would love the chance to care for you, like coworkers, neighbors, and those you've interacted with in your community. They may want to pick up deliveries for you, bring you your mail, help you with your phones and devices, or simply treat you special. *Let them.*

- **Paid caregivers:** If you have little to no personal support network, think about asking for help finding paid caregivers or a nursing facility. I see this quite often, and although almost everyone resists at first, in the end, they're so happy they asked for help.

  (Note: This can be hard financially—and I understand not everyone can afford a paid caregiver. At the end of the day, caregivers are the missing link in our health-care system, since some people truly can't afford them and don't have anyone to help. So what do they do? Sadly there is no good answer, except to try to work with the hospice company and apply for help.)

How to Have Difficult Conversations

We all naturally want to avoid talking about subjects that make us uncomfortable. I'm not sure that instinct ever serves us, but it definitely doesn't do any good at the end of life. Please try to talk about what you're facing with others. Your loved ones may be trying to tread lightly to save you discomfort or embarrassment. Give them an opening. They are looking to you for cues. You can let them know what topics are fair game . . . and most, if not all, of them should be. This may be the last chance you have to say the things you really want to say to each other.

Talk about Your Feelings

When we resist our feelings, they don't go away. When we embrace them, though, they lose their power to cause us suffering. If you're sad, denying it won't help you. If you're angry, refusing to admit it only makes the anger stronger. Face your feelings— first by feeling them yourself and then by talking about them with others. Not only does this create space for you, it also can make room for others to feel what they're feeling.

When you say, "I'm really scared," you make room for your partner to say they're scared, too.

When you admit to your child, "I'm so desperately sad to miss what's coming up in your life," you make room for your child to experience their sadness, too.

When you confess, "I am so angry that this is happening to me," you allow your loved ones to express and feel their own anger.

Now, there are a few caveats here. You're under no obligation to open up to people you don't feel safe with, such as family members who have a history of being abusive. Additionally, you want to be conscious of staying age-appropriate when talking about emotions with children. Lastly, I don't want to imply that you're responsible for other people's feelings. You're not. But when you start the conversation with the appropriate people, you give everyone permission to feel and to share. This can be an incredibly powerful thing. If you aren't sure how to go about this, a hospice social worker can help.

Talk about Dying

Be bold; talk about death. Most people don't want to, but when you do, when you push through your discomfort or fear, you'll find something extraordinary on the other side: peace. On my social media channels where I educate people about death and dying, I've received thousands of comments and messages from people telling me that learning more about the process of dying and being able to talk about it has eased their anxiety about death.

When you look death in the face, it loses its power to bully you. If your death has not yet been part of the conversation in your family or in your home, then your loved ones may not know it's okay to talk about it with you. Bring it up first, so they know you're okay with it, and when you do, don't sanitize it. Use all the d-words: *dying, death, dead, died.*

Death is happening to us all. You just have more information about *when* it might happen than most of us do. I've seen time and time again that those whose journey toward death has been the most peaceful are the ones who were *prepared* for it. They faced it. They talked about it. They felt it. They grieved it.

Talk about What's Unresolved (Maybe)

Are there relationships in your life that have unresolved problems? Do you need to make amends with anyone? Is there something you still need to say to someone? Consider talking about what's unresolved.

Now, I'm not suggesting you need to right every wrong, seek out every person you've ever harmed, or even hold accountable those who've hurt you. I just mean that you have a unique opportunity to face what you may have ignored until now.

If you feel that a situation will only end in more chaos and harm, then just let it go. But if you sense that there's a real possibility that you or someone else might experience freedom, go for it.

If you need help sorting it all out, use all the resources you've built so far: trusted counselors (spiritual or otherwise), loved ones, friends, the hospice social worker or chaplain, and/or anyone else you've invited to help you on your end-of-life journey.

Advance Care Planning

In this book, we're talking about the end of life. For many people, the end-of-life journey begins with a hospitalization. Say you have cancer, but you're receiving chemotherapy and don't necessarily expect to die for another few years. But maybe you get an infection, and the chemo has weakened your immune system so much that you can't fight it off on your own. You go to the hospital, where they try to treat the infection. Depending on all sorts of different factors, you may recover fully from the infection and continue receiving cancer treatment, or you may enter hospice, or anything in between.

Situations like this can be very chaotic, and it can be difficult for the patient or their family to make decisions on the fly. If the patient is unable to communicate their own desires and hasn't expressed those desires ahead of time, their family members might not know what they want. (If the patient hasn't given much thought to a scenario like this beforehand, they themselves might not even be sure what they want.)

That's where advance care planning comes in. Advance care planning lets patients and their loved ones review their options and make decisions about medical care ahead of time, so that if an emergency arises, the patient's wishes are clear and loved ones don't have to make agonizing choices under difficult conditions.

Here are some of the most common life-extending measures used in hospitals, which you'll want to consider when advance care planning:

- **Hydration:** As I discussed in chapter 4, intravenous (IV) fluid is given through the veins.

- **Nutrition:** A nasogastric (NG) or nasoduodenal (ND) tube is a flexible tube inserted through the nose to deliver nutrition into the stomach or intestines, respectively. Total parenteral nutrition (TPN) delivers nutrition through the veins.

- **Medications:** These include vasoconstrictors to keep a patient's blood pressure up or IV medications to help the patient's heartbeat.

- **Ventilator:** This machine assists the patient with breathing.

- **Extracorporeal membrane oxygenation (ECMO) machine:** Also known as a "heart-lung machine," this device is used in critical-care situations to oxygenate blood outside the body. This allows the blood to bypass the heart and lungs so these organs can rest and heal.

- **Continuous renal replacement therapy (CRRT):** This type of dialysis machine is used twenty-four hours a day to slowly and continuously clean out waste products and fluid from the patient.

If you're dying, the decision about what life-saving measures you might want to receive is yours. I encourage you to speak with your doctor about which ones might be right for you. But as you're making those decisions about what kind of medical care you want to receive, do consider your unique situation: what illness you have, how your illness is progressing, and if these measures truly will be beneficial. Think through the possible outcomes ahead of time, and consider situations in which you might choose to reject these measures.

You'll also want to think about what you want when it comes to resuscitation. Whether you're at home or in a hospital, you might face a medical emergency in which your heart and/or lungs stop working and you will die without immediate intervention. Your two main choices when it comes to resuscitation are as follows:

- **Full code:** This means that when a person stops breathing or their heart stops beating, everything possible—including chest compressions, intubation, and defibrillation—is used to keep the person alive.

- **DNR:** DNR means "do not resuscitate." Choosing this option does not mean that the person won't receive any care while they're still alive. Patients who choose DNR ahead of time still may choose to have surgery and other treatments, but if their heart or lungs stop working, they would prefer to die naturally, without resuscitation. This might be the right choice for someone who has multiple chronic illnesses and wants to die a natural death.

If you've gotten your medical education from television and movies—which many of us have—it can look like the heroic measures of a doctor or paramedic have the power to bring someone back from the dead. If you're strong and healthy, that may be true. But statistically speaking, most people do not survive resuscitation. And if you're terminally ill, your body is already dying, whether or not you're resuscitated. If you've insisted on CPR, intubation, and tube feeds, the inevitable outcome is that eventually your family will have to make the grueling decision to take you off the machines that are keeping you alive.

The most important thing is that you and your family have these conversations early. This gives the person who is dying the opportunity to say, for example, "At the end, I don't want a feeding tube." And, down the line, it gives the family the opportunity to say, "Mom told us what she wants, and she didn't want a feeding tube." You can see how making that decision early in the process of dying will serve you well. It's easier to reject a feeding tube at the beginning than it is to allow one and then have to have it removed. The end result may be the same—having no feeding tube at the time of death—but it can be easier on both the patient and the family when the decision is already made because you discussed it early.

Advance Care Documents

There are two main kinds of legal documents used to express a patient's advance care planning wishes in the United States: advance directives filled out by the patient and medical orders filled out by a physician. The required forms and terminology can vary from state to state, but I'll give you a simple overview so you have a general idea of where to start, what to choose for yourself, and how to make it all legal.

Advance Directives

The phrase *advance directive*, or *advance health-care directive*, can be used as an umbrella term for any instructions a patient gives, written or spoken, about the care they want at the end of life if they're not able to make their own decisions. In the United States, "advance directive" usually refers to a specific legal document filled out by the patient, stating their desires for care in a few key areas. These areas are as follows:

- **Power of attorney for health care:** This section lets you designate a person, such as your spouse, parent, or child, to make medical decisions for you if you're unable to make them yourself.

- **Health-care instructions:** This is where you state whether you want life-extending measures like those described above, what kind of pain medication you want or don't want, and any other medical instructions you want to give.

- **Organ donation:** This section lets you indicate whether or not you want your organs to be donated in the event of your death.

- **Primary physician:** This lets you list a specific doctor as your primary physician.

You can find advance directive templates for your state by searching online. You generally don't need a lawyer to fill out the form, but you likely will need to get it notarized or signed by witnesses.

Physician Orders

Whereas an advance directive is written by the patient, physician orders for life-sustaining treatment (POLST) is a medical order written by a doctor and intended as a complement to the advance directive. Also known as medical orders for life-sustaining treatment (MOLST) or medical orders for scope of treatment (MOST), this document communicates directly to health-care providers what you do and do not want in a medical emergency.

Most POLST forms cover three main questions:

1. If needed, do you want to be resuscitated with CPR?

2. If needed, do you want to be intubated to get air into your lungs?

3. If needed, do you want a feeding tube?

There may be additional questions, such as whether you want to be transferred to a hospital and whether you want antibiotics for an infection.

If you're potentially interested in a POLST, visit polst.org or talk to your doctor about filling one out.

What I Want at the End of My Life

If I end up needing hospice care at the end of my life, here's what I would want:

1. Do not give me IV fluids at the end of my life. This won't change the outcome; I still will die. Because my body will no longer be able to process fluids, they will do more harm than good.

2. Do not give me a feeding tube at the end of my life. This won't change the outcome; I still will die. Although nutrition was important to keep me healthy throughout life, it does not serve me well at the end of life.

3. Do not intubate me. I don't want to be kept alive hooked up to machines.

4. Do not administer CPR at the end of my life. If I'm forty-four and in relatively good health, by all means, give me CPR if I need it. But if I've lived a long life and am dying, do not give me CPR.

5. Be honest. Tell me the truth. I gain nothing by you hiding information from me, and I benefit from having all the facts.

6. Keep me clean, safe, and comfortable. Change me if I'm wet, turn me intermittently, and keep my mouth moist with sponges dipped in ice-cold water.

7. Speak as if I am fully present. Assume that I can hear you and understand you, even if I can't tell you what's on my mind.

8. Have *The Office* playing at all times. This one's self-explanatory.

Things to Do before You Die

After Reggie was diagnosed with bile duct cancer, his physical decline was rapid. His wife and two daughters scrambled to bring in hospice care for the last three weeks of his life. They kept Reggie comfortable and spent time being with him and caring for him. But when Reggie died, things quickly became difficult.

Reggie had handled *all* the family finances for four decades. His wife was a very capable woman, but he'd never shared much with her about their financial affairs. So although in theory her daughters could have helped her navigate banks, credit card companies, and investments, in practice, Reggie hadn't left a paper trail. Or a digital trail. Not only did his family not know the relevant passwords, they didn't even know where various accounts might be held.

In Reggie's situation, he truly didn't have time to prepare his affairs before he died. But if you've received a terminal diagnosis, I encourage you to do what you can, with help from your family, in order to *help your family*.

Here's a list to help you get started with some of the tasks that will make your death easier for your loved ones. If you have any questions as you consider these end-of-life decisions, ask your hospice social worker for guidance.

1. **Choose a mortuary.** Before you need it, choose a mortuary. If you shop around and contact a few places, you can make the best choice. If you wait, they may hike the prices because they know it's a last-minute situation. So plan ahead.

    First step: *Ask your hospice agency to recommend a mortuary, ask others in your community, or look at reviews online.*

2. **Share your passwords.** Something as simple as printing a list of the passwords you use—for your phone, email, banking, credit cards, investments, social media, and so on—can be a huge gift to your family after you're gone.

   Here are some passwords to share now:
   - *Phone (both the password to unlock your phone and the password for the account you use to pay your phone bill)*
   - *Desktop and/or laptop*
   - *Master password for your online password manager (such as LastPass)*
   - *Email*
   - *All social media accounts*
   - *All bank accounts and credit cards (online passwords, verbal passwords to give over the phone on customer service calls, and PINs)*
   - *Investment accounts, retirement accounts, insurance accounts, etc.*
   - *Utilities (gas, electric, water, etc.)*

   First step: *Communicate to someone you trust where your passwords are and how to access them.*

3. **Draft a will.** A will is a legal document in which you express your wishes about what you want for your property—money, home, car, investments, etc.—after you are gone. It also specifies what care you want for any minor children. I can't stress enough how important it is

to create a will. If you don't have one, it becomes much more difficult for loved ones to settle your affairs after you're gone.

First step: *Contact an attorney who specializes in estate planning.*

4. **Get your financial affairs in order.** If you're the person who's dying, handle as much of your financial business as you can. If you need help, enlist someone.

   Also, consider establishing a trust. A trust is an agreement that empowers a third party, the "trustee," to manage assets on behalf of a beneficiary or beneficiaries. One benefit of creating a trust is that the beneficiaries can gain access to these assets more quickly than if they were transferred using a will. There also may be fewer taxes after your death.

   First step: *Contact a financial adviser and/or estate planning lawyer who can tell you how to best protect and distribute your assets.*

5. **Execute an advance directive.** As discussed earlier in this chapter, an advance directive is a legally binding document indicating what you do and do not want in terms of medical treatments. After you've completed the advance directive, make sure someone knows where it is.

   First step: *You can find an advance directive template online. It's best to have this notarized, especially if the family isn't in agreement.*

6. **Appoint someone to be your financial power of attorney.** When you appoint someone to be your durable power of attorney for your finances, you create a document appointing this person to make financial decisions for you when you're no longer able to make them yourself. This person is then able to sign a check in your name, sign your tax returns, and even buy and sell property that belongs to you. These provisions can be drafted so that they're effective immediately, or they can be worded so that they go into effect when you are incapacitated. (Sometimes a single document can delegate authority over both medical and financial decisions.)

   First step: *Put this information in your will or advance directive. (See step 3 or 5.)*

7. **Appoint someone to be your medical power of attorney.** When you appoint someone to be your durable power of attorney for health care, you create a document appointing this person to make health-care decisions for you when you're no longer able to make them yourself. A power of attorney for health care is different from a financial power of attorney in that it *only* becomes effective when you are incapacitated. (Sometimes a single document can delegate authority over both medical and financial decisions.)

   First step: *Put this information in your advance directive. (See step 5.)*

8. **Consider how you'd like your body to be treated.** Do you want to be buried? Do you want to be cremated? If cremated, do you want your remains to be kept or scattered? Where?

   First step: *Discuss your wishes with family or friends. Also write them down.*

9. **Consider how you'd like your obituary to read.** This task is optional, but if you want to offer input on your obituary, share that with your loved ones. For example, you may prefer to use the word *children* rather than *stepchildren*. If you want to help shape the content or language around the way you're remembered, let your loved ones know.

   First step: *Write down, or enlist someone to write down, what matters most to you in terms of how you're remembered.*

10. **Consider how you'd like to be memorialized.** This task is also optional, but many people find it meaningful. How would you like your life to be remembered, honored, or celebrated? Do you want your loved ones to remember you at a funeral service? A memorial service? Do you want to participate in a celebration of life while you're still living? There are two ways to approach these possibilities.

    The first is for you to be very specific about the way that you would like to be remembered. If you're a person of faith, you may want to choose readings, songs, and prayers in advance. If you'd like to join the party and hear all the nice things people have to say about you, then plan a celebration of life while you're still living.

The second way to approach a service of remembrance is to leave it in the hands of those who will be remembering you. For example, would you feel comfortable turning it over to your siblings or another family member? If you believe that a service of remembrance is meant for those who are gathering, you may choose to let your loved ones decide how they'll honor your life.

If this is something that you have opinions about, consider some of these questions:

- *Do you want a funeral service in a church, temple, synagogue, or another religious gathering place?*
- *Who would you like to officiate the service?*
- *Do you want your body to be present at the service?*
- *If your body is on display, what do you want it to look like? What clothing, makeup, and jewelry do you want to wear?*
- *What would you like to be included in the service?*
- *Do you want a memorial service (maybe at a park, restaurant, or bar)?*
- *Do you want a celebration of life? A going-away party?*

First step: *Write down what you'd like, and share it with someone you trust.*

I know all of this can sound overwhelming. Admittedly, it's a lot. But it's a little like exercising. When taking your first run, it can feel like it's *too much*. But each run after that gets easier. Just like going on one jog is the first step, making one phone call to a lawyer is the first step. When you do that, you're in motion. The lawyer knows what needs to happen next. Or the hospice agency knows what needs to happen next. Or your clergyperson knows what needs to happen next. You begin by taking that first step to set it all in motion.

You can do this. Remember, to live fully, you need to plan for death.

Chapter 8

Advice for Caregivers

In chapter 1, I mentioned the Netflix series *From Scratch*, in which Amy's husband, Lino, is dying from cancer.

In one episode, we see Amy's family gathered around a table in the backyard, looking at their calendars and trying to figure out how to provide care for Amy, Lino, and their seven-year-old daughter. They've busied themselves with tasks they can do, but no one's talking about the fact that Lino is in the process of dying. After squaring away responsibilities for the upcoming two weeks, someone asks, "What about next month?"

Cautiously, Amy's sister Zora asks, "Are we sure we should be looking that far ahead?"

With anxiety in her voice, her stepmother, Maxine, asks, "Zora, what are you saying?"

Amy's father interjects, with kindness, "The doctors haven't given up on him. Lino's beat this thing before. He'll do it again."

Maxine adds, "He's got all these people pulling for him. And I started a prayer chain back home."

Amy's mother jumps in: "And once he's stable, there's a treatment I read about in Mexico."

This family that's deeply committed to their dying loved one is facing a moment that many families face.

As Amy's family cares for Lino in the United States, his mother, back home in Italy, prays for her son. When Lino is speaking to his mom on the phone, he hands it to Amy, who steps out of the room.

His mother confides in Amy, "Last night I dreamt of the Blessed Mother. She told me Lino was being called home. She was—"

Amy interrupts her mother-in-law to say, "Filomena, I know you're scared, but please, I can't hear that right now."

This often is how it happens in real life, too.

The cheerleader says, "He's beat it before. He'll do it again."

The religious one says, "I started a prayer chain."

The optimist says, "There's a treatment I read about."

The denier says, "I can't hear that right now."

And yet Amy's sister, Zora, was facing reality squarely. Reluctantly, she admits, "He just doesn't seem to be getting better."

Fighting for life is what we were built to do. Throughout human history, those who are wired to fight for survival have lived long enough to pass on their genes to future generations, and the human race has continued to flourish. Whether it's warding off the threat of a wild animal or pursuing the most effective treatments to fight a disease, I call this the *fighting mentality*. In many cases throughout life, it serves us well. But when a person is near the end of life, the fighting mentality is no longer helpful.

Continuing toxic treatments that will not restore any kind of quality of life can cause sickness and fatigue.

Forcing food and hydration can cause pneumonia, fluid overload, and respiratory distress.

Resisting what's coming can cause the person to be physically and emotionally agitated.

Persistent denial can rob the person who is dying of a peaceful death. Knowing what I know, when I'm with people who are dying, it's difficult to hear family members who are stuck in the fighting mentality. We can move this a different way.

Let Go of the Fighting Mentality

When you're in that fighting mentality as a caregiver, you want the person you love to return to being the healthy individual you once knew. So you fight—possibly literally fighting with the person who's dying—to get there.

The fighting mentality can be expressed in many different ways, but the kinds of messages I've heard sound a lot like the cheerleader, the religious one, the optimist, and the denier:

"Don't think that way."

"Pray for a miracle."

"You're a fighter."

"Don't give up."

"You never know. God could heal you."

"We're not going to give up on you."

"You're going to get better."

I understand we often don't know what to say, so we say

things to try to inspire pep, energy, hope, and victory. But it's usually not helpful. We're likely in a room where the person in front of us is, or will soon be, dying. When we're stuck in the fighting mentality, we're resisting what is actually happening. When we do that, we may be robbing the person who is dying of their right to be in the present moment and accept what is happening to them. What if we keep hoping *and* we fully prepare ourselves for death? What if both can exist alongside each other?

The critical question, of course, is: how long do we "fight" to survive? When do we accept that the person we love is terminal? I wish I could offer you a magic formula, but of course, every situation is unique. The best advice I can offer you is to pay attention. Listen to the medical professionals who are caring for the person who is dying. Listen to the person who is dying. If they're resisting outwardly, notice what their body is saying.

Be realistic, and accept what is happening. The most beautiful, peaceful deaths I've witnessed have happened when both the person who is dying and those around them have accepted the reality of the death that is happening.

Let Your Loved One Be Your Guide

If you're a caregiver, let the person who's dying be the boss. I want to emphasize this for *you*, the caregiver or other loved one of the person who is dying. Across the board, the more we let the dying person's body be the guide, the better they'll feel and the more peacefully they'll die. Caregivers need to hear this as

When to Continue Treatment

When medical treatments can restore the dying person to full health, they should be used.

When there's a likely chance that medical treatments can offer your loved one a longer life that can be well lived, they should be used.

When doctors have run out of treatment options and death from the disease is imminent, accept that death is coming. Then help the dying person live each day as well as they can.

When your loved one is in the active stage of dying, accept what's happening. Help prepare them, and yourself, for a peaceful death.

much as the person who is dying. If the body wants to sleep, it should sleep. If the body isn't hungry, it doesn't have to eat.

I understand that your natural inclination is to make sure the person you love is well hydrated, well fed, and well rested. You may want to line up visitors to make sure the person who is dying isn't lonely. You may feel cautious about offering too many pain medications. I want to relieve you of these very well-intentioned impulses. Although they come from a good place, let them go.

Our goal at the end of life is for the person who is dying to live as well as they can. If he needs more pain relief, advocate for that. If she wants a greasy cheeseburger, get her a greasy cheeseburger. If she turns her head when you try to offer her water, stop offering her water. Everybody is different, and every body is different. Let the dying person guide you in how to take care of them. Even if some of these choices feel counterintuitive after a lifetime of trying to pursue healthy living, at the end of life, they may be *exactly* the right choices.

The truth is, things in your loved one's life have changed. The rules at the end of life are different from the rules at other stages of life because the goal has changed. This moment is unique.

The rules at the end of life are different from the rules at other stages of life because the goal has changed.

Don't waste time arguing about food, drink, exercise, sleep, or medications. If you respect your loved one's wishes in these respects, you're not being a bad daughter or son. You're not doing something wrong. You're not hastening your loved one's death. If they don't want to eat, they don't have to. You don't have to stop them from sleeping "too much." You're not making them die quicker. It's their body, they truly know what they need, and you can—and should—respect their choices. Honor your loved one who is dying by allowing them to guide the process in all the ways they're able. This may help them, and you, find peace.

When Your Loved One Is Alert and Oriented

When your loved one is alert and oriented, they're the captain of the ship. When they make their wishes known, you have the opportunity and obligation to honor them. If you resist, you're likely just causing unnecessary stress. You may even be causing suffering. If, instead, you respect the dying person's wishes about how they want to live, you give them an extraordinary gift and ease the burden on you both.

When Your Loved One Is No Longer Alert and Oriented

When your loved one is no longer alert and oriented, pay attention to what their *body* is telling you. If you lift a spoonful of food to their mouth and they receive it well and swallow it easily, continue to feed them. If they close their mouth shut, making it difficult to feed them, don't feed them. Take a break and maybe try again in a few hours. Even if they can't communicate verbally, you can trust that their body 100 percent knows what it needs and wants. If you're ever in doubt, call your hospice team; they'll be happy to discuss the appropriate care with you.

Don't Force It

Maureen, in her early seventies, was caring for her father as he died. Despite the fact that the ninety-seven-year-old man did not want to get out of bed, Maureen dragged him up and forced him to walk to the kitchen and back every afternoon. When he refused to eat, she badgered him to drink Ensure, which he also didn't want. In her conversations with me, Maureen insisted that her father needed IV nutrition and hydration, even though I explained that it wouldn't serve him well. When she noticed a bit of redness on his buttock, Maureen set her alarm to go off every two hours throughout the night so she could turn him in his bed. While I appreciate the intentionality with which Maureen was caring for her father, she was doing *too much*. Her father would have been better served if she'd just let him be.

I had a lot to say about forced feeding and hydration in chapter 4, so I'll be brief here: it breaks my heart when I see caregivers prying open the mouth of a person who doesn't want to eat and forcing food into them. (I see this a lot with family members who think they're being helpful, but I've also seen it from paid caregivers who were actually *trained* to force food into patients.) Sometimes providers will argue that although the dying person has stopped eating, they're not yet at the end of life. I would answer, "If they're not eating, then *yes, they are* at the end of life." Stopping eating is one of the signs that a person is nearing death. I understand the impulse to make your loved one eat and drink, but I encourage you to resist.

There are medical reasons not to force food and water—it can, for example, lead to aspiration pneumonia. (This is especially important to keep in mind with patients who have diseases like Parkinson's or dementia, in which the body eventually loses the ability to swallow.) But there also are just human-to-human reasons. When you ignore the wants and needs of the person who is dying, you're squandering the time you have remaining together. Why spend that time struggling and arguing?

Clearing the Bedside Table

When I walked into Maz's bedroom, I noticed that his bedside table was filled with various drinks. Straws were sticking out of untouched glasses of water, orange juice, a bottle of Ensure, and a melting smoothie. The table was also crowded with all kinds of foods and snacks.

Maz's wife was sitting at his side, encouraging him to eat. "Just take three more bites," she urged, touching his lips with a spoonful of soup.

Appearing tired and clearly uninterested in food, Maz kept his mouth closed and turned away his head.

His wife pressed: "You need to keep up your strength."

With the very best of intentions, she was trying to help her husband. The problem was that she *wasn't* helping. When you're dying a natural death, your body naturally will shut down the mechanism that makes you feel hungry or thirsty because nutrition is no longer needed. Much more important than providing nourishment is to make sure that the dying person is clean, safe, and comfortable.

Once I explained this to Maz's wife, she understood. Together we cleared the bedside table of all the snacks and drinks she'd piled up there. This relieved not only her anxiety but Maz's as well, and they then had space to just be together during his last days.

It's a waste of time and energy. Even when someone is nonverbal, if they refuse to accept food, honor that wish. When you allow the person who is dying to be the guide of their own death journey, you make a peaceful death possible for them.

Don't Worry about "Bad" Habits

Sometimes, in the homes I visit, I notice caregivers put a lot of energy into behavior management. Specifically, I see this when the dying person is making choices that the caregiver doesn't approve of. Sometimes this may be as benign as eating too many cookies. Sometimes it's more serious.

If you're a caregiver, I want to relieve you of the impulse to control the behavior of your loved one who is dying. Ultimately, this isn't your journey; it's theirs. If, in the future, you have the opportunity to know your life is coming to an end, when you're the person who is dying, you'll get to call the shots. But for now, the person who's dying gets to do it.

The person who is dying should be allowed to make their own choices. You may not agree with those choices, but to the degree that they can express their wishes, the person who is dying has the right to do any and all of the following:

- Drink alcohol

- Smoke cigarettes or marijuana

- Eat foods high in sugar and fat

- Receive enough medication to control pain

"But Julie," you may be saying, "letting the person who's dying run the show doesn't feel right to me. She can't eat donuts because she has heart disease!"

Or, "The reason he's in this mess is that his drinking caused cirrhosis of the liver!"

Or, "She has lung cancer *because* of smoking!"

I know, I know. All I can suggest is that this is the time to let that go. When someone is at the end of life, it's not the moment to fight for what would have been healthy in another stage of life. It's not the moment to bully the person into eliminating their unhealthy habits. It usually doesn't work anyway. This is the point of surrender. The person who is dying surrenders to the disease that is taking their life, and you're going to surrender to the fact that they will die from that disease. I also encourage you to surrender your desire to control the person who is dying.

Do you have to hang around and watch them suck in the nicotine? No. Do you need to watch as they take a swig from the flask? No. But do let the person who is dying make those personal choices for themselves.

Don't Be Afraid of Pain Relief

Let's be clear about what is and what is not your role as your loved one journeys toward death. My hope is that as you own what's yours and release what's not, your load will be lightened. As a caregiver, you play an important role in the life of your loved one who is dying. They should be steering the ship, but you're on the crew. One of the most important ways you can support them is by helping manage their pain (if they have pain).

I once heard a patient ask a paid home health aide for morphine, and the aide gave her Tylenol instead, insisting it was all she needed. I kept my cool and quietly pulled aside the aide to gently educate her about why the patient deserved to receive the morphine. Shockingly, she continued to resist, assuring me that Tylenol would do the trick. I'm not sure if this caregiver had a moral issue with morphine, was poorly trained, or was simply apathetic to her patient's needs, but there was simply no getting through to her.

I finally just said, "You do not have a say in this. The patient is the only person with a say in this. The medication was ordered by the doctor. She's saying she wants it. That's what she gets. If you cannot give this patient the medications she needs, then you do not need to be her caregiver. Do you understand?"

I then administered the morphine to the patient, and, of course, it relieved her pain.

I wish that this type of event, when a caregiver refuses pain medicine to a person who is dying, was an isolated incident. Sadly, it's not. My heart breaks when caregivers deny the person who is dying the pain medications that have been prescribed by a doctor.

I do not believe that most caregivers are trying to be cruel. Rather, I think they have misconceptions or misunderstandings about morphine and other pain relievers, such as the following:

- They fear that their loved one will become addicted.

- They're afraid of delivering too much medication.

- They're afraid of killing the patient with morphine.

- They believe that giving morphine means that the dying person has "given up."

- They believe that morphine is only appropriate in the final hours of life.

- They believe that if morphine is offered "too soon," it won't work later when the pain increases even more.

- They fear side effects that can include nausea, constipation, or drowsiness.

I understand that there may be a lot that's unknown. But the reality is that morphine and other pain relievers prescribed by a doctor are safe and effective ways to treat pain. By using them, you help the dying person who may be in pain be the guide.

Honoring Medication Choices

At the end of life, patients often will choose to take the medications that make them feel better and reject the ones that don't. For example, they might refuse vitamins, cholesterol medications, or heart medications, but may choose to take their pain relief medication. Honor their choices.

Talk about Death

I often hear family members dismissing the experience of the person who is dying. It can sound a variety of ways:

"Don't say stuff like that, Dad. You're not going to die."

"Don't talk about how much you love me. You're not going to die."

"I don't want to learn how to take care of the garden because you're not going to die."

I know this can be hard, but you do the person who is dying a disservice when you don't let them speak their truth. They know that they're dying, and they deserve space to talk about it.

Is it comfortable talking about death? Rarely. Is it a way to honor and care for the person who is dying? Absolutely. It's always time to talk about death. Talk about it when you're sick. Talk about it when you're not sick. Talk about it at the Thanksgiving dinner table. There's never a time not to talk about death. Please acknowledge the experience of the dying person and the reality of their condition.

It's always time to talk about death.

Evaluating Your Loved One's Decline

One of the hardest things at the end of life is giving up control. Our bodies naturally decline, and we no longer can perform many of the functions we always have taken for granted. We may find ourselves unable to do simple things like comb our hair or make our way to the bathroom. Because we're so used to living independent lives, many of us struggle to ask for the help we suddenly need. On top of that, our ability to communicate our needs may have declined as well.

On the flip side, as caregivers, we now may find ourselves in the position of having to take responsibility for our loved ones' most personal needs. This can be awkward for some people, especially when the dying person is not communicating their needs, intentionally or not.

As a hospice nurse, one of my duties during a visit is to ensure that your loved one is clean, safe, and comfortable. I, too, have run into stubborn or incommunicative patients who refuse care. I always reassure them, saying kindly but with authority, "I just have to check to make sure you're clean, safe, and comfortable."

Most times, everything is just fine, but sometimes I find that the patient does have an issue, such as bed sores or diaper rash due to bowel and bladder incontinence.

When I speak with the family, they usually have no idea what's going on because "Mom assured us she was taking care of herself" or "Dad has always been so independent."

I'm not laying any blame here; caregiving is a big job. Changing family roles can be hard to navigate. We don't want to overstep our bounds, so sometimes family members won't realize that their loved one has let bathing, grooming, or going to the bathroom slide.

This doesn't have to be a complicated situation. There are six basic areas you can pay attention to, which health-care professionals refer to as activities of daily living (ADLs). They are as follows:

1. Ambulating or functional mobility

2. Feeding

3. Dressing

4. Personal hygiene, such as bathing, grooming, and brushing teeth

5. Continence, or the ability to control bladder and bowel function

6. Toileting, or the ability to get safely to and from the restroom, use it, and clean oneself properly

To evaluate whether a person needs assistance with any of these, simply ask: "Is my loved one able to remain clean, safe, and comfortable when executing this task?" If they're not, they will need help doing the task. If they're the sort of person who is resistant to help or reluctant to give up control of parts of their life, talk to them. It can feel awful to lose independence, but as caregivers, it's our job—and legal obligation—to keep our loved ones clean, safe, and comfortable.

And as always, if you're unsure about how to do any of this, talk to your hospice team. That's what they're there for.

Don't Do It All on Your Own

One of the best ways to help your loved one is to make sure that *you* have all the help you need. When the load feels really big, I want to encourage you to allow yourself to receive help. This can take different forms:

- **Accept help from people who offer.** Even if you think they can't or won't do it the way you'd do it, let them try. Even if it gives you a break for just a few hours a week. You need it—you need and deserve time to do something for yourself (or do nothing).

- **Ask for help from people who care.** Ask family, neighbors, friends, distant relatives, and members of your faith community for help. Be willing to say, "I'm drowning, and I need help. Let's come up with some ideas together."

- **Ask others to visit.** If you find yourself feeling upset that others aren't visiting your loved one, do something about it. There are a variety of reasons people stop visiting that often are complicated. I encourage you to ask directly for others to visit.

- **Receive respite care offered through hospice.** Your hospice provider may offer respite care. This means your loved one will temporarily stay in a care facility so that you can get a break. It may take some effort to organize, but it's worth it.

- **Pay for help, if you're able.** Not everyone can afford to pay for someone to help with their loved one's care, but consider that possibility if you can. You may find that others are willing to contribute to this cause as well. This is the time. Ask.

I understand and respect that you may *want* to do everything for your loved one. But you will be able to care for them more effectively if you also care for yourself by finding ways to rest and recharge. Accept help that is offered; ask for help if not offered.

Accept help that is offered;
ask for help if not offered.

Can Your Loved One Hear You?

Toward the very end of life, your loved one may not be conscious or lucid, and you may wonder if they even know you're there. You may wonder if the person who's dying can hear you when you speak to them.

"We're all here now, Dad."

"I love you, Mom."

"Whenever it's time, you can let go."

People who've been in medically induced comas sometimes report that they could intermittently hear doctors, nurses, and loved ones speaking. We can't say for sure if that's true in every situation, but it's entirely possible that, at the end of life, your loved one can hear you, even when they can no longer respond.

Science confirms this. According to researchers at the University of British Columbia, when sensors were placed in the brains of dying people, they showed that the hearing center of the brain was the very last part to shut down. This means that hearing is the last sense that we lose when we die. As a result, those of us who are around the person who is dying should behave as if *they can hear everything*. It's likely they can.

Just Be

Before I close this chapter, I want to say that taking care of someone at the end of life is one of the greatest acts of love a person can perform. Watching someone you love slowly die can be very hard, but you do it. To me, that's love in action. It makes my eyes well up each time I think about it.

As a caregiver, you're doing a lot. *I see you.* When you love someone who's dying, your impulse often can be to do this, do that, do the other thing, and then do some more. You want to care for the person you love, so you busy yourself with all the things. It's understandable why we shift into that mode, but I want to give you permission to make a different choice. When your loved one is dying, I encourage you to pause from your *doing* and focus on just *being*. Be with yourself, noticing what's going on inside you, and be with your loved one who is dying.

When you're up late at night, tossing and turning, your mind racing with anxious thoughts, remind yourself that your baseline is clean, safe, and comfortable. Once you've achieved that for your loved one, you really can let the rest go.

It may feel counterintuitive or even impossible to release doing in favor of being. But believe me when I say that this is what matters most to your loved one, and ultimately, it's what will matter most to you. What you're offering your loved one in terms of physical care is already priceless. Yes, your loved one needs you to do things for them at this moment because there is much they may not be able to do for themselves. However, I also encourage you to pause now and again from all your doing. Give yourself permission to *be* with the person you love. There is no greater gift you can give them or yourself.

Ideally, you'll have as much time as you want and need to just be with them while they're still lucid. Use this time to tell them how much you care for them. Let them know that you hear them and honor them. Listen to what they tell you. Share these moments.

There will always be a list of daily tasks that have to be accomplished. I encourage you to take time to pause from them and just spend time with your loved one. You won't regret it.

Chapter 9

Death with Dignity

I first met Miss Cynthia when I was doing her admission at her home. She was a fiercely independent woman who'd lived a rich, full life but had dealt with a lot of adversity. She'd battled chronic illnesses throughout her life, and at age seventy-four, she was diagnosed with advanced lung cancer. She went on hospice care when she was seventy-six.

Miss Cynthia didn't have family with her, but she did have a beautiful network of supportive friends. It was easy to see why: she was an absolute delight to be around. She was funny, cool, and thoughtful. She understood fully what was going on with her health and wasn't living in denial. When she began to need around-the-clock care, her amazing friend group took shifts spending time with her. When they couldn't, they paid for someone else to be there. These loved ones made sure she had everything she needed.

About a month after her admission to hospice, I got a call to go see Miss Cynthia. When I entered her room, I could see that she seemed comfortable and didn't appear to have any issues, so I was confused about why I'd been called.

As we chatted, she shared with me the ways she'd been declining. She was often in pain and was frequently short of breath. Knowing that she didn't have to be uncomfortable, I called the doctor to discuss the changes we could make with her medication to help with her symptoms. I was finishing up my visit when Miss Cynthia opened up about what was *really* bothering her. Since I'd first seen her, her functional status had declined as well. That meant she needed people to help her get out of bed, go to the bathroom, get changed, take a shower, and so on.

Miss Cynthia began crying quietly. Leaning in, I listened.

"You know," she explained, "I feel embarrassed."

"About what?" I asked.

"The biggest thing that's bothering me," she said, "is that I'm losing my independence. It's driving me nuts. I've been an independent woman my whole entire life. I'm super private. The fact that I have to have someone get food for me, or do this or that for me, is miserable. I hate it. I'm ready to go. I wish there was something I could take to let me die on my own terms."

At that moment, I knew I could tell Miss Cynthia about end-of-life medication. A number of states, including California, where I live and work, have "death with dignity" laws. This legislation allows eligible individuals to request and obtain medications from a doctor to end their life in a peaceful, dignified manner. Miss Cynthia had brought up the possibility of choosing death with dignity, and although I was not legally permitted to *suggest* it, once she *asked*, I was allowed to have the conversation and provide her with the very best information about medical aid in dying.

After explaining a bit of how it might work, I shared who she should contact about exploring the process further.

"Thank you so much," she gushed. "I feel like I have renewed hope. I'll look into it."

When I left Miss Cynthia's home that day, I knew I'd helped her. I'd truly connected with another human soul. Whether or not she chose to take end-of-life medication didn't matter to me; that was a choice for her to make, based on what was right for her. It had been an honor to have connected with her in an honest, true, and raw way.

Four weeks later, while I was in my car making notes after a patient visit, I received an email reporting that Miss Cynthia had died peacefully at home after taking the end-of-life medication. Now I was the one who was crying. She got what she wanted and needed. She exercised autonomy to choose the way she left this world, and I was able to help her with that.

Many of us have images in our minds of what an intentional death looks like. Maybe we've seen a movie in which a death row inmate is injected with a poison that ends his life. Or we may remember the headlines from when the then-controversial Dr. Jack Kevorkian—aka "Dr. Death"—was arrested and tried for helping a man with ALS die by physician-assisted suicide. Many have had these little tastes of what intentional deaths may be like, but I've found that very few people have a strong working knowledge of what death with dignity looks like in practice today.

Deaths like Miss Cynthia's are peaceful and beautiful, yet many people don't have the legal right or the access to supportive medical care they need to experience a peaceful death by ending their own lives with dignity. If you are someone who's in the process of dying, and you live in a place where this is an option, you have the right to explore the possibility.

Where Is Death with Dignity Legal?

Medical aid in dying is legal in some form in several countries around the world, including Australia, Austria, Belgium, Canada, Luxembourg, the Netherlands, New Zealand, Portugal, Spain, Switzerland, and parts of the United States. Within the United States, currently eleven states or districts allow it:

1. California
2. Colorado
3. Hawaii
4. Maine
5. Montana
6. New Jersey
7. New Mexico
8. Oregon
9. Vermont
10. Washington
11. Washington, DC

To learn more about which states have death with dignity legislation in place and which are considering it, visit deathwith dignity.org/states.

Who Qualifies?

Each state has important legislative measures in place to ensure that those who choose death with dignity are making the choice of their own free will, without being influenced or pressured by anyone else. These measures vary from state to state, but some common baseline requirements include the following:

- The person must be an adult over the age of eighteen.

- The person must have a terminal diagnosis with a prognosis of less than six months to live.

- The person must be a resident of the country or state in which they are seeking end-of-life medication.

- The person must be mentally capable.

- The person must be able to administer and ingest the medication independently.

There are other safeguards, as well, such as requiring an unbiased witness to the request or the approval of two physicians familiar with the patient's case. And of course the patient has the right to withdraw the request at any time; even if you get the medication, you can always change your mind and not take it.

The criterion that is most likely to disqualify those who would otherwise be eligible is the stipulation about being able to administer and ingest the medication independently. This means that people at the end of life with diseases like Parkinson's or dementia are unable to qualify when they're either physically or cognitively unable to perform these tasks.

<u>The Choice Is Yours Alone</u>

A few years ago, I was with Frank, a patient who was curious about taking end-of-life medication. As I began telling him about how it worked, his caregiver, who was in the next room, overheard us talking about it. Rushing in, she said, "No, no, no, no. He doesn't need that. He doesn't need that."

I paused the conversation and invited Frank's caregiver to speak in another room. "Listen," I said, "what's going on?"

I really loved this lady. She was a great caregiver. But I knew it was hard enough for Frank to ask me about it, and she was making it even harder for him to consider his options. When I gently explained to her that it was Frank's choice, she agreed with me, at first.

When I visited the next week, she told me, "I talked to Frank, and he said he was just lonely. He said he was in pain, and I promised to keep him out of pain. I said I'd take care of him and we'd pray more."

I explained to her that both of us needed to support him. I wouldn't try to persuade him to take the medication, and she wouldn't try to convince him *not* to take it. The choice would be his alone. We had to give him some grace by letting him decide and then supporting his choice.

In the end, Frank took the end-of-life medication and died peacefully in his home, surrounded by his loved ones.

How End-of-Life Medication Works

After the end-of-life-medication is secured in accordance with all state laws, the process goes like this:

1. **Anti-nausea medicine is consumed.** An hour before taking the end-of-life medication, the person who is dying takes two different anti-nausea medications to ensure they won't vomit up the end-of-life medication.

2. **The end-of-life medication is taken.** After waiting an hour, the person who is dying prepares the medication. The specifics of the medication vary by location, but in California, where I live and work, it comes as a powder in a small plastic bottle. The patient adds three ounces of water to the bottle, shakes it up, and drinks it quickly. (It's necessary to drink it quickly to ensure you consume the entire dose before you fall asleep.) I'm told the taste is bitter, so I suggest following it with just a spoonful of sorbet.

3. **Sleep.** Within three to five minutes, the person who consumed the medication will fall asleep.

4. **A peaceful death is experienced.** Soon after the person falls asleep, their body goes into the phase of actively dying. The person usually shows no signs of pain or distress, but there are signs that the body is actively dying. (See chapter 5 for more detail on these signs.) The dying process typically takes between forty-five minutes

and a few hours. If a hospice nurse is present, they will pronounce the patient legally dead.

You Get to Choose

When a person secures end-of-life medication, they need to let the hospice team know. The person who is dying gets to choose who is present and who is not; a hospice team member doesn't need to be physically there at the death, but they do need to be informed.

What Death with Dignity Looks Like

I recently sat with a patient before, during, and after he took end-of-life medication. Little else in my hospice career has felt so profound.

I sat with him until he was ready. First, he took the anti-nausea medicine. An hour later, it was time for the end-of-life medicine. As the nurse, I couldn't touch it. He mixed it up and then drank it quickly. Because it is time-sensitive, it does feel a little urgent. Once you drink it, there's no going back.

His loved ones were all around. They had already said their goodbyes and had a bunch of laughs prior to this, and they were all sharing their love with him. They all surrounded him, saying, "I love you. We're here for you."

After drinking the medication, he lay down and fell asleep within about three or four minutes. Then, during the next few minutes, his body began actively dying.

It's really that quick. You're awake, you drink the medication, you fall asleep three to five minutes later, and then you're actively dying.

At no time during this experience did this man look like he was scared or in pain or uncomfortable. His family surrounded him for the next forty-five minutes to an hour, until he died.

I was there just to witness and help explain what was happening: "Don't worry. These are normal changes in breathing." "Don't worry. We expect these terminal secretions and this sound. It's normal." If you're not used to seeing someone actively dying, you don't know what's normal, and these explanations really can help.

The experience of witnessing death with dignity is a heavy one. It's hard to watch someone say their goodbyes and then ingest the medication. It's hard to sit with the family as they wait for their loved one to die. It's sad. But it's also an honor to hold space and make the family feel safe and secure while sharing such a sacred moment. Typically, the level of love and support I get to see is unbelievable. I was glad to be there and count it a privilege to have shared that man's journey.

The Love I Witness

Before I close this chapter, I want to give you a glimpse of one more beautiful death.

"I'm going to take it on Sunday at two o'clock," Janie told me. "So walk me through how it works. You'll be here, right?"

Janie understood the inevitable outcome of her rapidly progressing disease and had decided to take end-of-life medication. I had been called in for a consult with her to tell her about the process. I was meeting her for the first time, and because I'm used to patients who are at the end of their lives often being lethargic, I was a bit taken aback by her vibrancy. She was alert. Oriented. Full of life. Her wife, Kylie, and her brother, Tom, joined us for the conversation we were having in the living room.

That Sunday, when I arrived at about 1:45 p.m., the door was unlocked. In many situations like this one, nurses aren't present, but Janie had expressed that she wanted me to be there at the end of her life, and I had agreed to join her. Inside, Janie's wife, brother, and best friend were cuddled up beside her in her bed. They'd been watching old home movies, singing, and laughing together.

Popping my head into the room, I said, "I'm here, but I don't want to intrude."

"No," Janie protested, "come on in!"

The atmosphere of life and vitality made the moment feel a little bit surreal.

"Did you take the anti-nausea med?" I asked, knowing she needed to take it one hour before consuming the end-of-life medication.

"Yeah," Janie said. "I took it around one o'clock."

A bit after two o'clock, Janie asked her brother to bring her some water so she could mix it with the medication. Setting it on the bedside table, he slipped into bed beside her. Janie's wife was on her other side. The friend who had joined them was behind Kylie. Janie was encircled in a cocoon of love. As her loved ones assured her that she was loved so very deeply, Janie took a sip of the bitter drink, wincing at the bad taste. Janie knew that despite the taste, she had to drink it quickly. Kylie handed her a teaspoon of her favorite sorbet as a chaser.

After Janie consumed what was in the glass, she lay down and smiled at her loved ones surrounding her. She said her "I love yous." Her people all lay down beside her, repeating, "I love you." "We're here for you." "I love you."

About a minute later, as if to ease the tension with a joke, Janie's wife said, "Bye!" in the breezy tone you might use when you're running to the grocery store. Everyone started laughing, including me.

Over the next several minutes, Janie's color changed, and she paled a bit. She *appeared* dead, but I knew she wasn't gone yet. After a few minutes she gasped a breath of air, which was her body's automatic response when in the process of actively dying.

"That's normal," I gently assured her crew.

They continued to hold Janie during the next hour as her body labored to let go of life. When I finally pronounced her officially dead, her loved ones peeled away one by one until just Kylie was left holding her.

Janie's death was one of the most beautiful things I've ever witnessed.

Chapter 10

Grief

The grief journey looks different for every individual. In the days and weeks and months surrounding the death of your loved one, you may notice that you are feeling a deep sense of sadness. This is normal. If you find yourself numb, not feeling any kinds of big emotions, that's normal as well. There's no right or wrong way to grieve. You might feel overwhelmed by the loss you've endured one day, and the next day you might be back to living your best life. The day after that, you may feel the sting of loss again. Not only is there no right or wrong way to grieve, there's no predicting the way your grief will unfold. It will be what it will be. Whatever you feel is the right thing to feel.

If you're the person with the terminal illness, the grief you feel can be an overwhelming and multilayered experience. Initially, you may grapple with shock and denial, struggling to accept the harsh reality of your prognosis. As the truth sinks in, profound sadness may set in as you mourn the life you had envisioned, filled with dreams and aspirations that may now remain unfulfilled. As the days pass, you might oscillate between feelings of anger and bargaining, questioning why this fate has befallen you and desperately seeking any potential reprieve. The fear of pain, suffering, and the unknown can intensify your grief, making you reflect on the moments you might miss in the future—milestones, gatherings, and cherished time with loved ones.

Yet amid the pain, you also may find moments of acceptance, when you can reflect on the life you have lived and the impact you have made on others. In this complex emotional journey, you may strive to find closure, make peace with your choices and decisions, and find a sense of purpose even in your final days. From my experience, those at the end of life who are willing to feel and acknowledge all they're feeling seem to have a more fulfilled life and more peaceful death. This chapter is meant to help guide you through the grief and other emotions you might feel surrounding the death process.

There's no right or wrong way to grieve.

I want to acknowledge that I am a hospice nurse, not a certified grief counselor, and I encourage those experiencing grief to seek professional support from trained experts in grief and bereavement (which hospice does offer). However, I have witnessed and supported many patients and families on their grief journey, and I have seen firsthand the immense depth and complexity of grief. In this chapter, I'll offer you the lessons I've learned about grief, rooted in compassion and empathy, drawing on my experience witnessing the raw emotions that arise during times of loss.

Anticipatory Grief

Jordan's father, Mel, was in his late eighties. When Mel was diagnosed with progressive supranuclear palsy (PSP), a degenerative neurological disease in the Parkinson's family, he still seemed very much like the man Jordan had always known. As his balance began to fail, Mel began using a wheelchair and sleeping in a hospital bed set up in the living room.

In the earliest months and years of his diagnosis, Jordan and Mel's relationship continued much as it had always been. But as Mel began to lose his cognitive abilities, he was no longer the quick-witted conversationalist he once was. During many conversations, he stayed mostly silent. He became even more removed at Friday family pizza night and during Jordan's frequent visits to the retirement facility where Mel was receiving care.

By the time Mel died, peacefully, with his wife holding his hand, five years had passed since his diagnosis. During those five years, Mel's family had been *grieving*. Although their patriarch was still alive, there were ways in which he ceased being there for them like he always had been. So the grief that descended when he died, which didn't at all feel overwhelming, was an extension of the grief that had been unfolding over five years.

When a loved one is taken suddenly in a way we never saw coming—by a stray bullet or a drunk driver, for example—our grief descends just as suddenly. But when our loved one has been given a terminal diagnosis, we *see* what's coming. Especially when we're the ones who accompany them on their journey toward death. When we can anticipate the imminent death of a loved one, our grieving process likely begins while they're alive.

When we can anticipate the imminent death
of a loved one, our grieving process likely
begins while they're alive.

Maybe a physical disease is slowly progressing. Or perhaps dementia has gradually been changing the person you know and love. In these cases, it's natural to begin to grieve while your loved one is still with you. Although you might think that spreading out the grief over a long period might lessen the sting, this kind of anticipatory grief—grieving *before* our loved one dies—can be very painful and very difficult. If you've experienced this "early" grieving, it's completely normal.

Anticipatory grief is an emotional journey that both a terminally ill person and their loved ones embark on as they confront the impending loss. For the individual facing the terminal illness, anticipatory grief can be an overwhelming experience as you grapple with the reality of your mortality and the uncertainty of what lies ahead. Feelings of sadness, fear, and anxiety may surface, along with a deep desire to make the most of your remaining time and leave a meaningful legacy. Coping with physical symptoms and treatments while simultaneously processing your emotions can be extremely challenging. Despite the pain, anticipatory grief also can open opportunities for personal growth, acceptance, and spiritual exploration, allowing the individual to find peace within themselves.

For the family of the terminally ill person, anticipatory grief can be equally profound and complex. You may experience a roller coaster of emotions, ranging from sadness and despair to anger and helplessness, as you witness the suffering of your loved one. Additionally, you may grapple with anticipatory grief over the impending loss of your roles in relationship to the dying person. Families often face the difficult task of balancing their own emotions and needs while providing care and support to their loved one. Communication becomes paramount during this time as family members need to express their feelings, fears, and hopes, fostering a sense of togetherness and understanding in the face of adversity.

During the process of anticipatory grief, the terminally ill person and their family may seek support from various sources. Hospice- or palliative-care teams can provide valuable assistance in managing physical symptoms and emotional distress, creating a compassionate environment for the person and their family. Counseling or therapy also can be beneficial in navigating the complex emotions and changes that arise during this period. Furthermore, support groups can offer a safe space for the family to connect with others who are going through similar experiences, fostering a sense of community and validation.

As anticipatory grief unfolds, cherished memories take on an even greater significance. Families often treasure the moments they share with their loved one, creating lasting memories to hold onto after their passing. These experiences can strengthen the family bond and become an essential part of the grieving process, offering comfort and solace in the weeks, months, and years to come. The anticipatory grief period also can be an opportunity for meaningful conversations about end-of-life wishes, allowing the terminally ill person to communicate their preferences for medical care and final arrangements, easing the burden on their family during the later stages of grief.

Ultimately, anticipatory grief is a unique and transformative experience that deeply affects both the terminally ill person and their family. It is a time of profound emotional growth, acceptance, and connection as they come together to support one another through one of life's most challenging transitions. Although the journey is undeniably painful, it also can be filled with moments of love, reflection, and a deep appreciation for the gift of life and the relationships that enrich it. Through open communication, professional support, and shared experiences, anticipatory grief can become a pathway to healing and finding peace amid the inevitable loss.

Grieving Together

If your loved one is dying, you're not the only one who's grieving. The person who's dying is experiencing their own grieving process as well. You can be instrumental in helping make room for their grief as well as yours. These conversations can be difficult, but I encourage you to have them.

Express Your Emotions

A gift that you can give your loved one is to be open to talking about hard things, like what they might be feeling about death and dying. One way to do that is to model the conversation by talking about what you're feeling.

If you're like a lot of people, you'd be just as happy *not* to talk about your feelings. But avoiding them doesn't mean they go away. In fact, the opposite is true. Psychiatrist and psychoanalyst Carl Jung famously said that what we resist persists. That means that when we refuse to feel our sadness, our fear, our anger— whether we avoid it, tamp it down, or numb it—it remains with us. When we allow ourselves to feel those feelings, they pass. Whether you're the person who is dying or you're accompanying a loved one who is dying, I encourage you to be brave. Allow your feelings. Express them:

"I'm afraid to die."

"I feel angry I'm going to lose you."

"When I think of a world without you, I feel so very sad."

I've been with hundreds and hundreds of people who are dying, and I've seen that the ones who are willing to express their feelings in some of these ways are the ones who have a more peaceful life and a more peaceful death. So even if it feels foreign to you, I encourage you to talk about what you're feeling.

Validate Your Loved One's Feelings

When the person who is dying expresses emotions that make you feel uncomfortable, like sadness, anger, or fear, it can be tempting to breeze past them or deny them. I get it. It can be uncomfortable to sit with someone who feels uncomfortable. We might feel the urge to minimize those legitimate feelings, saying things like this:

"Don't feel sad."

"Being angry isn't going to help anything."

"You don't have to be afraid."

"Why are you crying?"

We may think we're "making it better," but in reality, we're making it worse. There are few responses less helpful to a person who is hurting than to deny their feelings.

Instead, validate what they're feeling by saying things like this:

"I'm so sorry."

"That really sucks."

"I can't imagine what that must feel like."

If the person who's dying is crying, let them cry. (It's okay for you to cry, too.) If they're venting, let them vent. If they're overwhelmed by sadness, let them feel sad. Allow your loved one to experience their feelings. You let a person who is suffering feel seen, heard, and validated when you're able to reflect and affirm that what they're feeling—whatever it may be—is legitimate.

Practice Listening

As you try to make room for potentially tough conversations

with a dying loved one, I'd suggest *not* starting off with huge questions like "Are you afraid to die?" You probably won't get the most robust answer. Instead, you can set the stage for a good conversation by sharing your own feelings and then really *listening* to what the other person has to say.

Listening requires silence. Too often, when there's an awkward silence in a conversation, we'll jump in to fill the gap. It's okay to just listen and not say anything. When we allow silence, we make room for the other person to speak. That's a gift. Just listen. Don't interrupt. The less you talk, the more the other person may speak.

Caveat: All You Can Do Is Open the Door

Although I think it's very important to make space for conversations about death and dying, I never *force* someone to talk about it. The communication techniques I've suggested above assume that the person who is dying is capable of this kind of reflection, but they may not be. If the person didn't feel and honor his feelings throughout his life, if she avoided tricky topics, or if they had a lot of defenses to keep others out, then they may not have the tools to contemplate and discuss their feelings at the end of life. And that's okay. Allow the person to be who they are. All you can do is your part, which is to make space. It's messy. It just is.

If I was in this situation with a dying loved one who was not in touch with their emotions, I might simply model openness and vulnerability by saying, "I'm here to support you in any way that feels comfortable for you." I've opened the door, but if the other person doesn't walk through it, I can't—and don't want to—force them.

Complicated Emotions

When someone dies while under the care of a hospice team, I often have the opportunity to be with their family and other loved ones just after the person has died. The most common emotional reaction I see among them is this trifecta:

1. Relief

2. Shame and guilt

3. Sadness and grief

Caregivers often feel relief at the time of death because they've been—you've been!—doing the hard work of giving care that can be uncomfortable and exhausting and overwhelming. So it's completely natural to feel relief when a person dies. The wave of relief is often followed by shame and guilt. Caregivers might feel shame and guilt *because* they felt relief. Or because they weren't able to save their loved one from death. Or because they're alive while their loved one is not. Or for any other of a host of reasons. This, too, is natural. You may even experience that cycle of relief and shame and guilt more than once. Eventually, these initial emotions give way to sadness and grief.

So when your loved one dies, be very gentle with yourself. When you notice those feelings of relief, guilt, and sadness, I want you to tack on one more: *forgiveness*. I want you to forgive yourself for any feelings of shame about feeling a sense of relief after your loved one dies. These are the most normal responses! And you are not alone.

When I was seventeen, my best friend died suddenly. I remember getting the call and falling to my knees. I remember feeling shock and disbelief. I ran out my front door and through the yard, into the woods by my house, my mom yelling after me. I remember feeling like, if I could just run fast enough, I could run away from this, literally. I didn't want to believe what I'd just heard, so I ran. I can still feel the adrenaline even as I write this. The several weeks after her death are still a blur.

At the time, I knew nothing about loss. But looking back, I realize I experienced a variety of complicated emotions, and the way I grieved changed through the years. The main feeling that has lasted is guilt—guilt for surviving when she didn't, guilt for not being there the night she died, guilt for grieving too much or too little.

Recently, I was talking with a close friend about how I'd been thinking a lot lately about my friend who died, and that I was experiencing an unfamiliar feeling about her. I couldn't put my finger on it. I journaled about it that night, and as strange as this might sound, I realized that I felt resentment toward her. I was actually *mad* at her. After twenty years of her being gone, I finally let myself address the fact that before she died, I was mad at her—silly teenager stuff that we never addressed, but then she died. I carried around that anger for two decades and didn't even fully realize it. It feels embarrassing to admit because it was so silly. But acknowledging my anger and resentment set me free. I didn't even need a resolution; I just needed to allow myself to admit that I felt complex emotions I didn't expect to feel, including anger. I wept that night and woke up the next morning feeling so light and free.

Practice Self-Care

When your loved one has died, I urge you to be kind to yourself. Be gentle. Practice patience. Although there's no way of predicting what you'll feel and what you'll need, make room to notice. Rather than trying to quash them, *allow* your emotions to be expressed. If you feel lonely, reach out to someone who cares. Make room for your grief by taking time off work, if you can, or even spending some days away to process your loss and take time for yourself doing whatever it is that brings you comfort.

Here are some tried-and-true self-care methods, based on recommendations from grief experts:

- **Allow time for solitude.** Although community is important to the grieving process, it's also essential to create moments of alone time for introspection and reflection. Giving yourself time to process emotions, memories, and the impact of loss can aid the healing process.

- **Practice mindfulness.** Mindfulness techniques like simple meditation or breathing exercises can help you stay present with your emotions, acknowledge your grief without judgment, and cultivate a sense of inner calm.

- **Engage in physical activities.** Taking walks, doing yoga, or participating in some other form of exercise can provide a change of scenery, help you feel present in your body, and release endorphins, which act as natural mood lifters and stress reducers.

- **Journal.** Keeping a grief journal or otherwise expressing yourself through writing allows you to process your feelings, gain insight into your emotions, and find a sense of release and relief.

Remember that grief is a unique and personal journey, and some strategies may resonate differently with you. The important thing is that you prioritize taking care of yourself. You are worth it.

Journaling

As many of my social media followers know, I've been journaling on and off for the past twenty years. This practice has shaped the way I view myself and the world around me, and it has given me great relief during times of grief. You should journal in any way you feel comfortable, but if you have no idea where to start, here's how I do it.

I begin by directly addressing my higher power, who I choose to call God because that's what's easiest for me. You don't have to use *God*; the point is to write to something or someone you feel connected to—the universe, nature, or even the person you're grieving.

Then I write down everything, absolutely everything, in my heart and mind: the good, the bad, and the ugly. Sometimes, I'm writing so fast that it's barely legible. That's okay. I don't hide anything. It's a way of getting out everything that's inside me, emptying me onto the page. For me, it releases the grief.

Over the years, especially during my most desperate times, I believe I've heard back from God (or the universe or whoever). I've had many days when I was writing about my grief and felt I was receiving a beautiful message of love and support in response. This doesn't always happen, of course, and it's not why I journal, but when it does, it's a lovely benefit.

Grieve in Community

Although everyone's grief looks different, I want to caution you about the risk of isolating yourself after your loved one dies. In the United States, we live in a society that celebrates rugged individualism, but we weren't made for that. We were created to share life in community with others. We need a community around us as we grieve.

Here are a few ways to do that:

- **Connect with supportive family and friends.**
  Sharing feelings and memories with loved ones who

can listen empathetically can provide a sense of comfort, catharsis, and reassurance.

- **Attend grief support groups.** These groups provide a safe space to share experiences, feelings, and coping strategies with others who also are grieving. The sense of connection and understanding can be profoundly healing. If you can't find an in-person group near you, groups that meet online are available as well.

- **Create a memorial or tribute to your loved one.** This could take the form of a scrapbook, photo album, or even a tree planted in their memory. Engaging in these acts of remembrance can provide comfort and a sense of honoring your loved one's life. (This can be done in community with others who are mourning the same loss or on your own.)

What to Say to a Grieving Person

Not everyone will be the friend you need as you grieve. Some of the people in your life will be uncomfortable with grief. They might not acknowledge that you've endured a loss. They may even avoid you altogether due to their own discomfort.

Be the kind of friend to others who endure loss that you want them to be for you. Be *fully present.* Maybe you visit their home, or maybe you just sit together in the break room at work. After you say, "I'm so sorry," it's okay to then sit in silence. To stay present with their grief. To not fill the void with trite slogans or pep talks.

If you're not sure what to say to someone who has experienced a loss (or what not to say), the following table can give you some ideas.

THINGS TO SAY WHEN SOMEONE IS GRIEVING	THINGS *NOT* TO SAY WHEN SOMEONE IS GRIEVING
• "I heard about your mom. I'm so sorry."	• "At least he didn't suffer long."
• "What do you need right now? How can I be a friend?"	• "At least she had a long life."
	• "Be strong."
• "What is your favorite memory of your mom?"	• "God needed her in heaven more than we needed her here."
• "What does support look like to you?"	• "In time, you'll get over it."
• "Would you like to talk about it?"	• "Everything works together for good for those who love God."
• "There's no right way to feel. However you feel is okay."	• "He's in a better place."
• "I care."	• "There's a reason for everything."
• "I don't know how you feel, but I'm here to listen."	• "I know how you feel."
• "I remember how excited your dad was when you became a mom."	• Nothing.

Professional Help

As we've discussed, grief is individual and unpredictable. You may feel blindsided by intense emotions, oddly numb, or anywhere in between. Regardless of what you're feeling, if you've lost a loved one, you probably can benefit from seeing a grief counselor. Professional guidance can help you navigate the complexities of grief, provide coping strategies, and offer a safe and confidential space to process your emotions.

If your loved one died while receiving hospice care, the hospice company will provide you and the family grief or bereavement support for up to a year after your loved one has died. Please use it. And check out the Resources section in the back of this book for more books, organizations, and websites to help you on your grief journey.

Into the Future

As time goes on, your grief will evolve. Most people say they never fully stop mourning a loved one, but the grief ebbs and flows, and eventually they become more at peace with the loss.

Earlier in this chapter, I told the story of how my best friend died suddenly when I was seventeen. In the twenty years I've been grieving my beautiful friend, my feelings and actions have changed many times. In the beginning, I needed to be around friends who also were grieving, so we could reminisce and talk about our friend. I needed to visit her parents' house and see her room. I needed to miss school and rest. I needed to visit the cemetery where she was buried.

As the years passed, I needed other things. I connected with her in nature. I grieved and healed through journaling. I had many years of counseling. Throughout the years, I would have revelations about my grief that would free me a little more. As I described earlier, I'm still discovering new emotions two decades after her death.

Time didn't make my grief go away, but it did transform it. I still feel a profound, rich connection with my friend, but I also can move forward in my life without the heavy burden of fresh grief. You never forget a loved one who dies. You never stop loving or missing them. But eventually, over time, the burden becomes lighter.

Nothing to Fear

When I started in hospice, I wasn't at all sure what to expect. I knew I was going to be able to advocate for people who were dying. I hoped I would be able to make a difference in people's lives by helping them die better. What I didn't expect was what it would do to me. I get to see love in action nearly every day of my life. If I sometimes witness the opposite, too, it only serves to make the love I see even brighter. It has changed me. I no longer fear death, and because of that, I'm more prepared for life.

If there's one idea I want you to take away from this book, it's this: our bodies are built to die. They know how to do it. The more we can understand that, accept that, and prepare for our death, the better we'll live and the more peacefully we'll die. It doesn't matter if you have thirty days left to live or thirty years. We're all dying. Some people have more information about when that's going to happen, but it's going to happen to all of us eventually.

I've been present at many deaths. I've seen peaceful deaths and deaths that were a struggle. In nearly every death that was a struggle, there was a moment when things could have turned. There was always a moment when the dying person (if conscious and aware) or their loved ones could have chosen to accept what was happening, could have let go of resistance, and surrendered to what was. They could have stopped fighting an imaginary war against one of the greatest gifts we're given: a peaceful and natural death. They could have let go of the tension from this constant battle that wasted the days and hours they had left. Instead, rooms were filled with stress and anxiety and then grief and regret.

On the other hand, in every peaceful, natural death I've witnessed, there was an overwhelming outpouring of love. Families who listened to their dying loved ones were having better relationships with them. Conscious or not, dying people who were being allowed to die were less agitated, suffered less, and in many cases actually lived longer. The simple act of letting go, of allowing nature to take its course, of hearing for the first time everything that was being said to each other, created love as if out of thin air.

None of us *mean* for life to get away from us. We want to believe that we'll always be healthy. We resist thinking about death. But death is an essential part of life. It comes to our parents, it comes to our friends, and it comes to us. By ignoring it, we miss out on a huge, beautiful part of our existence.

We die the way we lived. Be intentional about both. Let death into your life. Talk about it with your loved ones. Don't leave them guessing about how you want to die. Don't wait for a terminal diagnosis. Do it now. Your death will be better because of it—and so will your life.

A Note to Hospice Nurses

In one TikTok video, a content creator who's a nurse gets into his car after a shift at the hospital and basically has a meltdown. I've never been tagged so many times as I was on his video! I clearly remember leaving countless shifts at the hospital when I worked as an ICU nurse feeling just like this guy did. I'd hold myself together during work and then I'd have a complete mental breakdown when it ended. I often sobbed, and if I wasn't sobbing, it was because, in that moment, I was dead inside. Completely detached from reality. I'm sure that different care providers reach this breaking point for different reasons. In my case, it was because I felt devastated by how we were allowing people to die (or keeping them "alive") in the ICU. I knew that there had to be a better way, but I didn't yet know what it was.

So even though this book is primarily written for people who are on hospice and their loved ones, I wanted to take a few pages to directly address hospice nurses or people thinking about becoming hospice nurses.

My path to freedom was to leave the hospital setting and begin my journey as a hospice nurse, but I know that yours may be different. But I see you. I see what you face. And here's the advice I can offer you.

Take Care of Yourself

Something that I wish I had learned sooner in my nursing career was to protect my wellness—especially when I was working in a hospital, but even now as a hospice nurse. In both settings, there are a lot of demands on you. Most days I adore my work as a hospice nurse, but there are also days or weeks that can be pretty heavy. During those times, I feel the sadness. I feel the gravity of the situations families are facing, and I feel deeply for them. I see their sadness. Their fear. Their fatigue. Their courage.

There is always a lot of work to be done, and if you don't pause to take care of yourself, you'll get weighed down by burnout. Your supervisor, whether that's a nurse manager or a hospice administrator, wants and needs you to do as much as possible, but if you get burned out, you won't be able to do anything. (And if you're hoping your manager will hire another nurse like they probably need to, ask yourself: if you continue to say yes to stretching yourself thin and they get everything they need from you, why would they hire someone else?)

You know what the stressors are in your unique situation. But here are a few strategies to consider as you think about what self-care looks like for you:

- *Leave after eight or twelve hours, at the end of your shift.*

- *Don't work overtime.*

- *Don't pick up extra shifts.*

- *Say no to things you don't want to do or can't do because of time restraints.*

- *Stand up for yourself if your place of work is asking you to do more than what's humanly possible in an eight- or twelve-hour shift.*

Will there be pressure on you to give and give and give? Absolutely. Is there an unspoken message that if you take care of yourself first you're not a "team player"? Certainly. If you take some of these steps to guard your own health and well-being, don't expect a lot of love from your supervisors.

Even though you're doing amazing work, caring for vulnerable individuals, you need to take care of you, too. You are worth it. If you aren't intentional about protecting yourself, no one else will be. When you protect your boundaries, you're not only doing right by yourself, you're also showing the rest of your team what it looks like to keep yourself healthy.

Be the Example

You already know this: it can be really hard for people to talk about death and dying. We also know that when people face reality as it is, they can live better and die better.

As a hospice nurse, you are such an important player in a family's story. When it comes to conversations around death and dying, you set the tone. If you're uncomfortable or sheepish about discussing it, you signal to a family that it's not something that can be discussed freely. But if you kindly and calmly name reality—"You are dying," "Your loved one is dying"—then you make room for everyone else to accept what is happening. When they're able to accept it, they can be prepared for a peaceful death rather than one that is fraught with resistance.

Here are some ways that you, as a hospice nurse, can model this:

- *Be comfortable talking about death and dying.*

- *Acknowledge that a person is dying. Don't be afraid to say the words* death *or* dying.

- *Be comfortable allowing yourself and others to express emotion.*

- *Talk openly about the patient's diagnosis, prognosis, and what to expect at the end of life.*

- *Openly ask and answer any difficult, possibly uncomfortable questions.*

In many homes, you'll encounter patients and family members who fear death. They don't want to talk about it. They don't want to admit that they are dying or a loved one is dying. They don't acknowledge that they or others might be feeling sad, angry, or fearful. But when you act as an example, embodying what it means to be a grounded, non-anxious person, you make room for others to do the same.

Final Encouragement

As a fellow hospice nurse, I want to remind you of the profound impact your work has on the lives of those we care for. What we do truly matters. We are granted the privilege of being present in some of the most sacred and meaningful moments of our patients' lives. In that space, we have the profound opportunity to help facilitate peaceful deaths and ensure that our patients' final journey is one of dignity and comfort.

It's not always easy, and sometimes we encounter resistance when providing necessary information. But even when faced with reluctance, we must remain steadfast in giving people the very best care and information they need. Our role is to be compassionate guides, supporting patients and their families through the emotional turbulence that comes with end-of-life care.

In the midst of caring for others, it's essential to take care of ourselves, too. Our well-being is vital because it directly impacts the quality of care we provide. Remember to find moments for self-care, and seek support when needed. We carry heavy emotions, and it's okay to lean on one another for strength and encouragement.

In our work, we communicate not just with words, but with all that we are. Our presence itself can provide solace and assurance to those facing their mortality. Let us be beacons of comfort, demonstrating through our actions and compassion that death need not be feared, but rather embraced as a part of life's sacred journey.

Know that you are capable and resilient. You've chosen a path of great significance and purpose. Embrace each day with courage and empathy, knowing that your presence as a hospice nurse profoundly impacts the lives of those you care for. You've got this, and together, we make a difference in the lives of others when they need it most. Thank you for all you've done and will continue to do.

Acknowledgments

I want to thank the following people, without whom this book would not have been possible:

Rich Cassone, an amazing writer who helped with the crafting of this book.

My nieces, Kortni and Kayci, who introduced me to TikTok, which opened up my life to a whole new journey beyond my wildest dreams.

Tim Sanford and Anastasia Arten, who encouraged me to educate on social media and always cheered me on.

Trinity McFadden, my literary agent, for believing in me and helping me along this journey.

Lauren O'Neal, Marian Lizzi, Christy Wagner, Sally Knapp, and the rest of the team at TarcherPerigee, for taking a chance on me, being so patient and warm, and helping me through this process.

Dr. Ana Cartmel, for being a shining example of a hospice doctor. She taught me everything I know.

My sister, Jill McFadden, for paving the way for me to follow my dreams and want the most out of life. My mom and dad, for always putting their kids first and supporting me. My brother—you are me, and I am you. I love you.

Jenny Phillips and Maggie Browne, for keeping me sane during my ICU days.

Shauna Jodon, who is always in my heart.

Jim Hopkins—just come in.

Chelsea Hogan, for showing me the path.

All my friends and family who supported me along the way—you know who you are. I love you.

And last but certainly not least, my TikTok community, for changing my life and hopefully changing others' lives, too!

Resources

Podcasts

End Well by Dr. Shoshana Ungerleider and Tracy Wheeler

Dr. Ungerleider is brilliant. She educates people about end-of-life care by welcoming to her podcast different guests who have a variety of perspectives.

It's OK That You're Not OK by Megan Devine

Grief expert and psychotherapist Megan Devine talks with people about their often invisible losses and what they've learned about being seen and supported in difficult times. Megan has such an incredible way of connecting with her listeners and understands grief so well.

The Waiting Room Revolution by Dr. Hsien Seow and Dr. Samantha Winemaker

Dr. Winemaker is my absolute favorite. She and Dr. Seow explain end-of-life care expertly and accessibly. Highly recommended for anyone with a serious illness.

Books

Gone from My Sight: The Dying Experience by Barbara Karnes

This little booklet by a renowned hospice nurse and end-of-life educator is a classic. It educates readers on the signs of death and dying during the last three months of a person's life when they're on hospice or palliative care.

It's OK That You're Not OK: Meeting Grief and Loss in a Culture That Doesn't Understand by Megan Devine

After hosting a podcast with the same name, Megan Devine, recognized as one of today's most insightful voices on grief, wrote this best-selling book that has helped thousands of people.

Hope for the Best, Plan for the Rest: 7 Keys for Navigating a Life-Changing Diagnosis by Dr. Samantha Winemaker and Dr. Hsien Seow

Written by the hosts of The Waiting Room Revolution *podcast, this book is a great reference for what to do when diagnosed with a life-limiting illness.*

Websites

Hospice Nurse Julie
hospicenursejulie.com; @HospiceNurseJulie on TikTok and YouTube
This is where I post videos to educate people on death and dying, tell stories about my life as a hospice nurse, and answer viewers' questions. You also can find me at the same handle on Instagram and Facebook.

American Hospice Foundation (AHF)
americanhospice.org
Although the AHF has ceased operations, its website's archived resources still provide valuable information related to hospice and grief support.

Death with Dignity
deathwithdignity.org
This website offers information and resources regarding medical aid in dying in the United States.

Dougy Center
dougy.org
Dougy Center specializes in grief support for children, teens, and families. They offer online resources, support groups, and educational materials related to grief and trauma.

GriefShare
griefshare.org
GriefShare provides grief support groups, resources, and videos for individuals who have experienced loss, including hospice-related deaths.

Hospice Foundation of America (HFA)
hospicefoundation.org
The HFA website offers educational resources, grief support, and information about coping with hospice-related loss.

Medicare
medicare.gov
Type the word hospice in the Medicare website's search function to find information on what hospice-related services they cover and how to access them.

National Hospice and Palliative Care Organization (NHPCO)
nhpco.org
The NHPCO website provides resources, support, and educational materials for individuals facing end-of-life care and grief.

National POLST

polst.org

This website can help you understand and plan a POLST or similar medical order.

Organizations

Compassion & Choices

compassionandchoices.org

This nonprofit offers a rich trove of information and resources on its website, on issues ranging from health-care equity to dementia end-of-life care.

The Compassionate Friends (TCF)

compassionatefriends.org

The Compassionate Friends is a national organization dedicated to supporting families who have experienced the death of a child. It has chapters throughout the country, offering in-person support group meetings.

End Well

endwellproject.org

Founded by Dr. Shoshana Ungerleider, who hosts the podcast of the same name, End Well is a nonprofit that aims to improve end-of-life care for everyone.

Give a Mile

giveamile.org

This organization helps people who live at a distance get to be with their loved ones before they die by providing fully free flights.

Mettle Health

mettlehealth.com

Mettle Health fills in the gaps in the health-care system with personalized consultations that provide support and guidance for individuals and families facing health challenges.

The New Normal

www.thenewnormalcharity.com

This British organization offers free peer-to-peer support groups, online and in person, for people around the world.

Index

About the Author

Julie McFadden has been a nurse, first in the ICU and then in hospice/palliative care, since 2008. Her TikTok channel, which educates viewers about death and hospice care, has more than one million followers, and her work has been featured in media outlets including *Newsweek*, *USA Today*, *The Atlantic*, *Business Insider*, *People*, and *BuzzFeed*. You can find her on TikTok, Instagram, YouTube, and Facebook at @HospiceNurseJulie. She lives in Los Angeles, California.